I0104670

KNOWLEDGE

— IS —

P⬥WERFUL

The information you need when
fighting cancer

Knowledge Is Powerful - The information you need when fighting cancer
Copyright © 2018 Deb A. Kientop

All rights reserved. No part of this book may be reproduced (except for inclusion in reviews), disseminated or utilized in any form or by any means, electronic or mechanical, including photocopying, recording, or in any information storage and retrieval system, or the Internet/World Wide Web without written permission from the author or publisher.

Book design by:
Arbor Services, Inc.
www.arborservices.co/

Printed in the United States of America

Knowledge Is Powerful - The information you need when fighting cancer
Deb A. Kientop

1. Title 2. Author 3. Self-Help

Library of Congress Control Number: 2018905822
ISBN 13: 978-0-692-12351-5

KNOWLEDGE
— IS —
POWERFUL

The information you need when
fighting cancer

DEB A. KIENTOP

*This book is dedicated to the
memory of my mom.*

Contents

Acknowledgements

To my parents, whose wisdom, love, and support made me who I am today. Together you showed the world how life keeps going after a cancer diagnosis, and how important it is to live each day to the fullest. Dad, it was your love and devotion that allowed mom to fight until she couldn't any longer. Thank you for taking care of her.

I would like to thank Dr. Philip Breitfeld, Joyce Cleary and LeAnn Jackson, for their willingness to share their stories, and expertise to make the book better. Phil, thank you for always taking my calls, and sharing your medical perspective. Joyce, my B.B.E., thank you for support and mentoring over the last 20 years. LeAnn, thank you for sharing your story, your strength inspires me.

Above all I want to thank my husband, Steve, my biggest cheerleader, who reminded me every day that even if this book only made life easier for one person, it was worth it. And to my three boys, who encouraged me in spite of the time it took me away from them.

Last and not least, I would like to express my gratitude to the many people who saw me through this book; to all those who provided support, talked things over, read, wrote, offered comments, and assisted in the editing, proofreading and design.

Introduction

This all started when I was nineteen, a few days after I came home from my first year of college. I learned my mom had found a lump in her breast the month before and was scheduled to go to the hospital for a biopsy. I was shocked. My mind was spinning as my father and I accompanied Mom to her surgery the next week. All too soon, my dad and I heard the surgeon say the word "cancer." I remember walking down the hallway of the hospital with my folks, my mother being pushed in a wheelchair in front of me, and the walls starting to close in around me, my vision going to black, the breath catching in my chest.

What were we going to do? My mother had cancer. How could I possibly help her?

After the initial shock and tears, it was clear that my mom was prepared to fight for her life, and I was determined to support her in every way possible. I made a silent promise to live life with my folks with absolutely no regrets, and to put my life on hold for however long it took to get my mother through this. Through the long months of standing by my mom as she fought harder than I thought possible, I came to see that terrible summer as something that came into my life for a reason.

In the next semester I chose my path in college, ultimately graduating with a pharmacology degree. At present, I have worked in the field of oncology for twenty-five years. Along the way, I came to face my own cancer diagnosis at the age of twenty-nine and tried to support my oldest sister as she faced breast cancer and the difficult treatments that awaited her.

What I've learned is that the fight is never easy.

How many days did we have to wait for test results that often seemed to bring bad news? How would my dad and I keep up our brave faces as we sat with my mom through her chemotherapy? How often did we compare our fantastically normal life before mom got sick with our life post-cancer? How would we learn to live as cancer survivors? But my mother showed everyone around her that you could *live* with cancer. She was the very epitome of a person living life to the fullest, even when she was taken down by the disease years later.

Always a strong woman, my mom came to survive her initial cancer with a determination I had never seen her display before. She lived for almost fifteen years cancer free before her second diagnosis. She was alive to see my sisters and me get married, to see all her grandchildren born, and to spend numerous hours bowling, miniature golfing, fishing, and vacationing with our family. Even into the last few years of her life, when she was not feeling well at all, we were able to fulfill a longtime dream of my mother's: to vacation together, my mom and dad, my husband and me, and our three kids at Disney World.

My mom finally found peace in 2009.

Cancer came in, the worst visitor anyone could ever have in their life, but it did not beat her, or us.

One thing my mother said to me during her twenty years of battling cancer that I always keep close to my heart was, "I'm so thankful that I have you with me," with her next words, "What about everyone who doesn't have someone like you? Who helps them?"

This question hit me hard when Mom first said it during her cancer battle. It came sneaking its way into my mind even after she got better and I began to work in the field of oncology. It hit me hardest when her cancer metastasized (spread) during those last few years of her life. I continued to be one of my mother's supporters and became her all-around answer person for her treatments and even the clinical trials she would undergo. I'll admit, I didn't always like having the answers to her questions. Knowledge might be power, but it's not a comfort when you can pretty much calculate to the month how long your mother has left to live.

But my mother was right; there are indeed lots of people out there dealing with cancer who don't have somebody to help them. I have beaten back plenty of tears imagining the man or woman who has no family living close by, who doesn't have friends beyond maybe a few coworkers they share a morning coffee with; the person suffering in pain and fear keeping their diagnosis a secret; the man or woman who has to drive themselves to their chemo appointments, circling a parking lot in vain trying to find a parking space each time (just writing this last sentence gives me chills). Or the person who feels a little sicker each day, has no idea why, but has inadequate healthcare or none at all, and fears what they might be up against if they do scrape up the money to go in for that diagnosis that they can hardly afford.

My heart goes out to anybody without a somebody in their life to help them. I am cut to the quick thinking of anybody going through cancer alone. Fear will rock you to the core when you're given a diagnosis that brings you face-to-face with your mortality; dealing with it all alone is almost too much for me to think about.

Even with a full support system, surviving means dealing with the realities of life as you grow ever more tired, sick, scared, and sometimes absolutely hopeless with worry: worrying about your job during and after your treatments (mainly, will you still have a job?); worrying over how you will pay for your treatments, or surfing the minefield of insurance to pay for them; worrying about who is going to take care of the people taking care of you; worrying about who is going to translate all of those doctor's terms; worrying about finding at least a few foods that you can eat, when just the smell of food can make you sick; worrying over the legitimacy of cures you might be reading about and want to try; worrying about what your quality of life will be like as you continue with your treatment; worrying about what your life will look like now without a breast or having to stay on a specific medicine for the rest of your days. All these worries lead to questions.

Yes, there's a mountain of responsibilities to consider, and specific concerns meet each person differently. I try to never take this for granted even though I know many of the answers given my education, job, and experience. I know that there are plenty of resources available to answer the multitude of questions; plenty of federal, state, and even worldwide support groups ready to help; and the Internet is a great social sphere to find fellow cancer sufferers and survivors, but a lot of the information might be lacking or simply not applicable to any one person's specific situation.

In many cases, the cancer patient isn't up to looking for or hearing answers, doesn't want to think about or talk about their cancer today, and simply wants to have a worry-free afternoon.

It's that age-old concern of getting the right information at the right time and seeing if and how it applies to your particular set of circumstances. God knows, the one specific truth about cancer is that everyone's journey is different, regardless of how many of us share the same kind of cancer or undergo the same kind of treatment.

What I've set out to do with this book is to provide a road map for finding your individual path through the cancer maze. You can read the book from cover to cover, or you might find jumping forward or back to the chapters that deal directly with your current questions might work best for you. My goal is to cover enough topics clearly that you'll come to pick up this book again and again when other concerns and questions arise. You can scour these pages for inspiration when you are feeling low.

I just hope as you read this, in whatever way you do, that you are comforted, informed, and that your health continues to improve.

Within each chapter you'll find background information on a specific topic, subchapters that deal with other aspects of the topic, as well as suggested resources and places to go for additional help and support. I also pepper in anecdotes when I can from my own story when I think they are applicable. What I've mainly tried to do is keep my mind in two camps while writing. One, as the layman, scared to death over a recent cancer diagnosis, either for myself or a loved one I am caring for. Second, as a professional who has spent years with these terms and distinctions, sharing some sound information as simply and succinctly as I can.

Speaking of professionals . . . to give you a viewpoint that goes beyond mine, I have enlisted the help of three friends of mine who each have a unique relationship with cancer, all from a different professional and personal perspective: Joyce Emerson Cleary, LeAnn Jackson, and Philip P. Breitfeld.

I met Joyce almost twenty years ago in one of my earliest jobs within the pharmaceutical industry. We were working closely with oncologists throughout the United States, both of us hoping to find and develop new treatments for cancer. In addition to her strong relationships with physicians and researchers, Joyce has been actively involved in supporting cancer advocacy work through organizations such as the Leukemia and Lymphoma Society. Her perspective is invaluable.

LeAnn and I met shortly after my mom passed away, when I left my consulting work and went into the clinical research industry. When I heard her story, and everything that she and her family were going through as they fought cancer with her son Cameron, I felt a connection. She is passionate about working with organizations that support cancer patients and their families, including St. Baldrick's Foundation, and continues to work closely with pediatric oncologists in the development of new treatment options through clinical trials. LeAnn's tragedy of losing her son, being brought down into the depths of the worst circumstance a parent ever has to face, and how she not only survived but is helping others is an inspiration to me daily.

I met Phil about six years ago, when we were working in the clinical research industry. He trained and has spent much of his professional career as a pediatric hematologist/oncologist, diagnosing and treating kids who have cancer at medical centers such as Dana Farber and Duke University. He has personal experience in helping patients and families navigate a cancer diagnosis, and he understands the importance of clinical trials and research in the search for new treatments and cures. He, too, offers insights I could not.

I can't thank my three friends enough for helping me with this book. Their honesty, friendship, and professionalism are the icing on the cake as far as I am concerned, and you will come to appreciate each of their perspectives and the knowledge they come to impart. They weigh in initially in chapter 2, and then you will see them adding their opinions, anecdotes, and advice all throughout the book onward.

They say two heads are better than one, so why not four?

You will find a takeaway section at the end of each chapter—my attempt to pluck out the most pressing points of each section. For more information I've also included resource pages beginning after chapter 2 (chapter 1 is more or less my biography). In these resource pages I've printed the URLs, phone numbers, and brief descriptions of many great institutions, cancer care groups, research article libraries, and communities represented by online sites you can avail yourself of specific to the subject just covered. Please note: I give only a brief overview of these sources at the end of each chapter; at the end of this book you will find a more detailed accounting of them, delineated by subject.

It's my fervent wish that you won't need this book for too long a time and that you or the cancer patient you are taking care of gets well ASAP! But we can't ignore the realities of this illness and its treatment; some trying times are ahead for you in dealing with cancer. Flip ahead to the subject that's most pressing in your life presently. Open to the last page and jot down a few website addresses; scribble notes in the margins. Take comfort or warning from my personal trials. Whatever you need, I hope this book proves to be an invaluable resource to you as well as a comfort for what lies ahead for you and your loved ones.

I wish you all the very best of health.

Chapter 1

Mom to Melanoma

It was going to be a good summer. Just days back from my first (and if I do say so myself) wildly successful year at the University of Wisconsin, I was sincerely looking forward to seeing and relaxing with my friends and hanging with my mom and dad. Things couldn't have been better.

But you know how it goes—the best of times, the worst of times.

Unknown to me, my mom had found a lump in her breast a month before. She had gone in for a mammogram in February and got the all-clear, but from a self-exam in May, almost a month to the day before I came home from college, she had found a lump. My mother was proactive about her health and certainly on top of her breast exams and mammograms, which was understandable, seeing as all her female cousins on her mom's side had gotten breast cancer. Up to the age of forty-nine, though, mom had been cancer free.

Until that May.

In her calm fashion, my mother hadn't told my two sisters or me about finding the lump, certainly not me with my finals looming. My sister, the middle of us three girls, was finishing her last year of college and preparing to go away for her clinical training, and my eldest sister was working and living away from our home, so none of us knew of the recent developments in my mom's health, nor would my mother tell us. After finding the lump, my mother had gone in for a follow-up mammogram and ultrasound and then scheduled a biopsy surgery for the week after I got home. I came home and found out.

The word from the surgeon at this stage was that he was confident he wouldn't find anything alarming. My folks were pretty stoic about the whole thing, while I was doing my best to digest this sudden turn of events, unpack, and hold on to the surgeon's positivity. Mom was a year away from fifty. She had years and years to live, right? This couldn't be such dire news. She'd be OK, right?

What I didn't know, but would come to realize as the story played out, was that Mom and Dad had pretty much cried all this out before Mom's diagnosis, or at least had considered cancer as a fait accompli over the years given my mother's family history. Also, with my father being a nurse anesthetist, he was more knowledgeable than most about medicine. He understood many of the questions my mom had—not that he had all the answers when it came to something as specific as breast cancer—and he could at least talk things through with my mother with some scientific knowledge.

Yes, the news of what my mom found rocked our little house and would come to change all our lives forever, but my parents were taking it all a lot better than me. Remember, this was 1989. Procedures, drugs, the whole approach to cancer screening, diagnosis, and treatment were so different way back when. We tend to take for granted the swift progression of technology and scientific advances that have occurred in the past decade, but comparing those last few years of the eighties to what we enjoy now is like comparing the Stone Age to the Renaissance. I didn't even have the Internet at my disposal to look up the specifics of the biopsy procedure. All I knew was that my mother was going in for surgery, and my father and I would be there.

These days, breast biopsies can be done by a specialized radiologist in a clinic or hospital, and the patient waits an agonizing couple of days to get their results. For my mother, that day at the hospital, the surgeon removed a sample of the lump he had found in her breast, sent it down to pathology, and got his answer while my mother was recovering.

He wasn't as positive when he got the results.

My mom had breast cancer.

This is when I blacked out. I remember walking with my parents out of the hospital, Dad and I behind Mom as an orderly pushed her wheelchair, and I experienced the classic tunnel vision. I passed out upon the realization that my mother had CANCER! My world was suddenly falling apart. What did this mean? Could she actually die? We didn't yet know how bad it was or what her chances were; was there any treatment that had a chance of working?

I had heard a bit about my mom's cousin's cancers, but the disease had never directly impacted my parents, sisters, or me. Over the years since, in my professional and personal life I have become all too familiar with breast cancer, but back then, home from my first year of college, at nineteen years old, I was woefully ignorant of what was coming for us all.

There also seemed to be a strange view of breast cancer back then, and an unwillingness to even talk about it. Fortunately, things have changed, and the public is a lot more aware of and therefore sympathetic about all kinds of cancer, not just breast cancer. People are willing to share their stories now, even of how they undergo surgery to prevent breast cancer, like Angelina Jolie.

But back when my mom was diagnosed, people simply did not want to talk about breast cancer, or so it seemed. In fact, I recall going to church around that time—this would be well into my mother's chemo treatment—hearing a couple of ladies gossip that my mother must have done something terrible to bring this kind of cancer on herself. How that could be possible, I have no idea, but breast cancer elicited this kind of prejudice way back when. There was not only an ignorance of the disease, which is certainly not the layman's fault in any way, but for those women suffering from it, there was a stigmatization over it. Even though my mother could be a very private person, she was able to draw upon her own experience and advise a couple of her church friends through their own breast cancer diagnosis and treatment; she was not afraid to discuss it, that's for sure.

It's my opinion that cancer needs to be discussed, diagnosed, and dissected across the cultural landscape as much as it can be. Cancer is awful, I can state that unequivocally, but all cancer needs to be examined in equal measure to bring us closer to a cure or, at the very least, better treatment for the patient who has it.

The first of many soapbox moments you'll get from me.

That June, the surgeon went from finding cancer in my mother's breast tissue to performing a single mastectomy on her and finding that her cancer had spread to her lymph nodes. Each time my mom went into the operating room and the surgeon came out to report to us, it felt like everything got worse and worse. Talk about the guy being a harbinger of doom! That summer we'd come to walk on eggshells, afraid of what the next bad news would be. Since mom's cancer had spread to her lymph nodes, she needed to be put on chemo to blast away any of the disease that might have spread.

I pretty much walked around like a zombie through June, July, and August. My mother's cancer was on my mind all the time, essentially muting any fun I could have had that summer. I had never seen my mother sick, and this unnerved me. She was a strong, proud woman who did for us unselfishly; now we had to do for her, in ways I frankly was not ready for. If we hadn't been close before, and we certainly had been, my mother and I grew a lot closer during the time of her treatment.

My friends were there for me as best they could be, mostly trying to engage me in diversions. But their conversations, concerns, and desires began to seem trivial to me as I saw a life and death struggle unfolding in my home. They were eighteen and nineteen-year-olds, young women and men with budding social commitments and school responsibilities always looming; how could I expect any of my friends to even understand? It was summer, after all; their minds were on taking a break from school and having a good time.

When something like cancer or any life-threatening, chronic health condition is affecting you or a loved one, it can be hard to handle. Philip P. Breitfeld, who you will hear more from later, calls it a "life event" when someone is diagnosed with cancer. That is how big of an impact a cancer diagnosis can have on both the patient and their caregivers/family/friends. I remember waking up some mornings and for a brief few seconds being free and clear of the worry, before the realization came to me that, yes, Mom still had cancer and we were all still in the middle of it. It was like waking up to a bad dream, instead of waking from one. We lived in the shadow of this thing that had come to live with us and attack my mom.

Six weeks after her surgery, in mid-August, my mother began her chemo treatment. At the early stage of her treatments, nausea hit her hard. This was years before the anti-nausea drugs that we have presently, and I can recall exactly how the smell of something my father and I were cooking in the house could make my mother sick. Mom's sense of taste also left her that first month, and she couldn't enjoy food at all. If chemo/cancer patients need anything those first few months, it is to keep their strength up by eating regularly. Here again, cancer had come into our daily life in a most insidious way, in that we had to carefully choose what to cook and eat on a daily basis.

Then my mother suffered through another terrible side effect that I think bothered her more than she would say: she began to lose her hair. As bad as it is for a man to lose his hair through chemo, it is doubly worse, I feel, for a woman. With our usual Wisconsin winter coming in a few short months, my mother was going to be very cold indeed without her hair.

As far as what was on my mind, I was going to stay put for the foreseeable future. I couldn't see the point in returning to school; my courses, roommate, college life, any and all plans for my future seemed to have no purpose at that point. Who cared for college in light of my mom fighting for her life? I'd take care of my mom and dad and stay home.

At least this was my plan until my parents got wind of the idea.

They were not going to have my mother's cancer seep into their daughters' lives. While my older sisters had been around during the summer and they called to check in as much as they could, like me, they had important things that they had to attend to, simply to keep living their lives. My parents were determined that nothing would be put on hold. My middle sister was halfway across the U.S. undergoing her clinical rotation, and my oldest sister was working a few hours away from home. I would be entering my sophomore year, and although God knows my head wasn't on school anymore, my parents would not entertain the idea of me not going back. It wasn't even up for discussion.

My folks took me back to college at the end of August, with my dad and me walking my belongings from the car to the dorm while my mother sat on my bed and tried not to appear as sick as I knew she was feeling.

I had carried a 3.5-grade-point average my first year at the University of Wisconsin, but that first semester of my sophomore year my grades saw a downturn. As you can suspect, my mind was back home with my folks. I was returning home almost every weekend, and without a car on campus, this involved a three-hour bus ride each way. My roommate was complaining I wasn't around, (sorry to say, I didn't much listen to her griping), and even though I did manage to go to a few of my professors to tell them what was happening, I didn't care all that much for college. Really, what was the point?

At the end of September, my oldest sister called to tell me that my mom had been admitted to the hospital. The chemo my mother had been on had made her dangerously ill. I was three hours away, living in a dorm with a roommate who didn't get what I was going through, all that school craziness going on around me—and me worried as it was—and I get this news?

I was terrified for the couple of days that it took for the doctors to get things under control for my mom. They ended up switching my mother's chemo, putting her on something even stronger, which is closer to the drug that they use today. I realize now that this switch, my mom being given a stronger drug and one that made her feel even more ill, may have been the reason for her being as cancer free for as long as she would be. While it may sound crazy, I'm almost thankful that this all happened.

That was a harrowing time—stuck at school, imagining the worst, hoping for a phone call but fearing it at the same time.

Of course, whatever I was going through was nothing compared to what my mother suffered. That's the crazy thing about cancer for the caregiver or family member, and something I'd feel time and again and have to battle constantly. Sometimes you get so wrapped up in what you are feeling, so bowled over by the fear and a cloying feeling of impotence that you lose sight of the fact that the patient is suffering in ways you can't even conceive and sometimes fail to see. We are all just human. You do the best you can and try to learn each time what to do and say that can make the patient feel better, putting your own feelings on the back burner.

By my winter break, my mom seemed to be feeling some relief. Her nausea had died down and she had grown back enough of her hair that she didn't need those funky knit hats I had been sending her. With her on the mend, I would come to a revelation about college.

The day that I returned to school at the end of January for the start of my second sophomore semester, I opened my mailbox to find a flyer from the university's School of Pharmacy. They were offering a new major in pharmacology and toxicology. I was leaning toward a science degree of some kind, and I had already taken most of the prerequisite courses for this new major. Seeing as this was the semester I'd have to declare my major, it seemed the stars were aligning.

Hey, maybe I could even help find the cure for cancer.

Clearer headed than I'd been in some time (I certainly was not clearheaded during the semester that had just passed), my mind was on what I was going to do now that Mom was feeling better. After the Christmas holiday, the New Year seemed rich with possibilities.

It might have been serendipity (or maybe just some good karma finally coming my way after all my mother had been through) that saw me find and then jump into my new major. By my next year in college, I was well on my way and would come to graduate with a B.S. in pharmacology. My first job out of college was working as a lab technician in a cancer research lab for an amazingly knowledgeable and talented Nobel Prize–winning researcher. It felt great to be at least a small part of trying to find a cure for cancer.

Unfortunately, after my first year, my boss was diagnosed with cancer; what he had spent his life trying to fight, ultimately took his life. With his lab closing, and with the urging of my mom, I made the decision to go back to school for a business degree and found a job as a technician in a cancer clinic—the same clinic that my mom had been treated at. This at least helped me feel like I was still involved in fighting cancer. After a few years, I transitioned into working in the pharmaceutical industry where I had the opportunity to meet and work with expert oncologists throughout the United States. Eventually, I moved into the world of clinical research where I presently work as a senior director of oncology project management. I have now been in the oncology field some twenty-five years.

Beyond my mom's cancer prompting my college career path, I think I was destined for math and science. As a little kid, I can remember saying that I was going to be a marine biologist . . . seeing, of course, as Green Bay has so many waterways near it. My sisters have careers in science and medicine (chemical engineering and occupational therapy, respectively), and my father was a practicing nurse anesthetist at St. Vincent Hospital for thirty-four years. Maybe this was as much nurture as nature with me.

It's not that my parents were hammering home scientific study above all else. My sisters and I often remark that ours was an abnormally normal household. We grew up in a healthy, loving home. My parents were the greatest parents ever, and ours was a solid middle-class life. We went on family vacations, had plenty of extended family around us who we often saw, and we enjoyed a great life all around.

Beyond the normal interplay and yes, I suppose at times, a teensy bit of drama from three girls growing up under one roof, there really wasn't ever and still isn't any rivalry or weird push and pull of personalities between my sisters and me. I can't say we see one another all that often, but I am close to them and their families, as they are to me and mine. My dad is still alive, and at eighty-one is an active, happy guy, beyond missing my mother, of course.

My older sister just completed chemotherapy and surgery a little over a year ago for her breast cancer, and even though we live far away from each other, I tried to help as much as I could with her concerns and treatment.

Just another reminder that cancer doesn't discriminate and changes the lives of everyone it touches.

⊙❈❈◎

I married when I was twenty-five, and four years later, a year shy of my thirtieth, with no kids yet, I had my first personal encounter with cancer. My mother had been cancer free for a decade, and there wasn't hide nor hair of the disease in my immediate vicinity for a good long time. Mom went in for her regular checkups, eventually stretching from three months to six in their frequency the longer she was cancer free. We had all been trying to live the typical each-day-to-the-fullest, as people often get reminded to do after a loved one, or they themselves, go through something life threatening. My work was good, my marriage wonderful, family healthy, and then . . .

I remember it clearly. It was the week before Christmas 1999. I had gone to the dermatologist to see about a spot I had noticed changing color on my lower back. This was how it had been for me all during my teenage years. I am fair-skinned and one of those people who has moles, lucky me. The dermatologist assured me that he could remove the odd-looking mole and there should be nothing to worry about. There hadn't been concerns with any of my moles before, so for me this was routine. They would "scrape" the mole to minimize damage and send it out to be tested, just to be sure. Even though they always tested as abnormal ("dysplastic" is the medical term), none of my moles had ever proven to be anything serious.

Here again, though, was another doctor showing too much confidence for his own good.

Four days later the nurse from that dermatologist's office called—his nurse, not the doctor!—to tell me the doctor had been wrong. I had melanoma. Skin cancer.

The rug of life was pulled out from under me. There are a couple of different types of skin cancer, but melanoma is the most dangerous and can be deadly. First, I called my husband, and then I called my mom. She left work to come sit with me until my husband could make it home. Clutching her, I simply reacted. By the time my husband came home later that day, my head was clearing. I wasn't calm, per se, but I slowly began marshaling a plan of action.

How could I, constantly preaching that getting-out-in-front-of-cancer attitude, not be the conductor on my own train now when it was pulling into cancer town? I could do this! I could take control in the way I always advised others to. If anything, I was the perfect person for the job of helping me through this.

First, given my job, I was much more knowledgeable about cancer by this point in my life. I was light years away from the scraps I knew back when my mom had cancer. With the personal ethos I had been living, "knowledge is power," I took it upon myself to apply what I knew and use it to my advantage. Second, I felt my job demanded that I be proactive. And last . . . I was mad. The dermatologist had made his nurse tell me. He couldn't even pick up the phone himself to deliver this terrible news? And that call had been brief, the nurse hanging up after a, "We will call you back to tell you what the next step is." As far as I was concerned, this was no way to treat a patient, especially someone to whom you have just delivered such dire news. Next step? I'll show you next step, I thought. I was going to find out, and right then, exactly what the next step was, and I was going to take it!

I made the decisions for *my* health. I was willing, able, and really, who else was going to make these decisions better than me? I was luckier than most in that I had a wealth of education to call upon, and I wasn't afraid to use it. Sure, when you learn the stuff you do, you never think how you might be applying it; I never thought that I'd end up being the patient I'd come to advise. But such was the case that I could, and would, damn well help myself now.

Calling a plastic surgeon the very next day, I set up my appointment, and we discussed how we'd be proceeding. He talked me through exactly what he would be doing, I asked questions (yes, just like I advise you to later), then I reached out to one of the oncologists that I used to work for and asked questions of him. I learned from my ex-boss that if any cancer was found during the surgery that the plastic surgeon did, I might need more treatment. So, I prepared myself for that eventuality as well, not because I am a fatalist, but because I wanted to be ready for that *next step* and act as proactively as possible to whatever the outcome of my surgery was.

By the time the dermatologist did get back to me two days later (yeah, he called me this time, not his nurse) to tell me his plan and about the plastic surgeon *he* had picked, I told him what we were going to do and what plastic surgeon I was going to use.

The facts of melanoma, not many of which I knew at that time (but facts I came to learn quickly) were that there weren't too many drugs or treatments touching that particular cancer at that time. Simply put, if you were diagnosed at a later stage with the disease, there weren't a lot of effective treatments, and a patient might be looking at something as low as only a 20% survival rate. This is definitely an area where great progress has been made over the last ten years, and there are new treatments available that provide real hope for remission. Unfortunately, these were not available when I was diagnosed. I was not yet thirty, and in my darkest thoughts I could now imagine my life over, never having had kids and dying way too young.

Luckily, I *was* diagnosed early. The plastic surgeon, a doctor who was involved with surgical treatment of skin cancer, managed to take a "wide excision" to make sure there wasn't any remaining cancer, which there wasn't. And even though I have had plenty of moles biopsied since, luckily, I have remained cancer free all these years.

Fast forward to just a year ago, and once again I took the bull by the horns. Given my family history, I know I have as high as a one-in-three chance of developing breast cancer, and possibly soon. So, I elected to have a double mastectomy. As you can imagine, there was more than a little back and forth between my doctor and me about my plans. Even though I had met with a genetic counselor who had mapped out my family history and helped me understand the results of my genetic testing and what my likely risk of developing breast cancer was, the surgeon initially disagreed with me. Because I did not have a known genetic mutation like BRCA 1 or BRCA2 (although I do have a few "variants of unknown significance"), she felt there was no reason to go in and cut my healthy tissue. Her recommendation was to follow a high-risk screening protocol, which would require yearly MRIs in addition to my mammograms, and to take anti-estrogen medication. I had already had abnormal mammograms and multiple biopsies (all negative), and I didn't want to live my life in fear any longer. I was adamant about what I was going to do for my health.

In the somewhat conservative, small population of Green Bay (small in comparison to other big cities), a woman volunteering to have a double mastectomy when no cancer is present is not common, not by a long shot

. . . just think about the press Angelina Jolie got when she revealed she had undergone the same surgery. But again, *I* decided. *I* was in control. *I* knew the double mastectomy was the best way to assure my continued good health. I have kids now, I am very fond of living life my life, and I want to be around for many more years to come.

I like to consider myself a smart woman. I know what the research shows and I know my chances. I certainly respect the opinion of health-care professionals, and I didn't want to provoke any kind of adversarial relationship between my doctor and me (especially with the one who was going to be doing surgery on me), but I knew what I wanted. I had explored my options fully, with my scientific acumen in fact, and knew that what I was doing was best for my health. (For the record: my insurance provider agreed with me.)

I talked it out with the surgeon. To her credit, every surgery carries some risk, and this is not a small procedure that should be rushed into by anyone. Some things cannot be undone.

It's also a generational thing, I think, as much as it is a personal consideration. As you can see in my mom's story alone, the passage of time brings us deeper knowledge—the impact of genetics and family history, better drugs and treatments, evolution in personal assumptions and considerations as the culture slips and slides through the years. My mother had one breast removed and never went in for reconstructive surgery, as this was never on her radar. She simply wore a prosthetic for the rest of her life and later, after her second mastectomy, my mother often went without her prosthetic altogether. For me, certainly my health came first, but after my surgery, I opted to take a two-stage approach for reconstruction. My busy schedule saw the two procedures stretching out to eight months between my first surgery and my second, although they normally wouldn't take so long to be finished.

From my mom's cancer to my sister's—from my melanoma to my preventive mastectomy, and even my reconstruction—the point I feel needs making here is: It's your health. Act on it, for it, and to better it, always. Ask questions. Delve into options. Explore as much information on what's happening with your specific disease and its current treatments as possible. If you are too weak or simply too upset to clear your head enough to make informed decisions or even research what you need, enlist those around you—friends and family who you know are going to be in this for the long haul with you—and together seek out the information you need. Constantly weigh what you learn against other facts, and grab as much as you are able from as many sources as you can. Stick to scientifically sound research and leave no stone unturned.

Ultimately, you need to take as much control as you can in this fight for your life.

Takeaways

- When you receive a cancer diagnosis, whether you are the one stricken or a family/friend of the patient, your world is going to change right quick. Start writing down the questions you have, and what your concerns and fears are. Perhaps you'll find answers or resources in this book that will help you.
- While you may never have a clear understanding of why you developed cancer, it's important to talk with your doctor about possible causes, in case there is something you can do to help yourself or other family members.

- Take control of your health and your healthcare. Take well-thought-out opinions, weigh options, listen, and learn as best you can, but in the end, you need to take control of your own health.

Chapter 2

Building Your Healthcare Team

OK, you have cancer.

I was initially devastated from what my dermatologist found. In that first rush of fear, I quickly thought my life was over. I was overcome with the absolute finality of hearing the word cancer applied to me. But I recovered quickly enough—after crying in my mom's arms for the afternoon—and did what I needed to do. I had been through my mother's cancer, and I was working in the medical field. I had a lot more knowledge than the common person. My survival scientific smarts kicked in, and I got to what I had to get to.

I may not be able to help you with that shock, but I can give you questions to ask and put you on the path to people who can answer them for you.

In the following chapters, I will take us down that dark road of the types of cancer that exist, exploring the one you have in more detail, and then its specific treatments. I know you are scared about what's currently attacking your good cells, and we will come to the specifics, I promise. But for right here and now, let's get into how best to build your healthcare team with people you trust. You could see this as a march into battle, where you'll need to amass the best troops around you. How you come to tackle the next few months depends greatly on the choices you make right now. While the family members and friends who go on this ride with you are surely a blessing, I think I can probably assume that they aren't prepared to answer the multitude of concerns springing up in your head, the first of which has got to be . . . choosing a doctor.

Choosing a doctor will be one of the most important decisions, if not the most important decision, you'll come to make. **Diagnosis, treatment, during, and further preventive care later on** will come from your doctor's influence and suggestion. You need to find someone you trust here, someone who will answer your questions—all your questions—as you will be looking for the medical professional who will provide the support that you need to make the quality of your life the best it can be during what might well be the hardest fight of your life. You likely will have to make some difficult decisions ahead, will have some terribly frank and personal conversations, and will experience some highly emotional moments.

It could be a long road back to good health, and the doctor you choose should be someone you can work closely with for quite a while.

As I explained at the outset, everyone makes their cancer journey in a wholly personal way, and no two people are alike in how they deal with this life event. Every patient is different in what they want from their healthcare professionals. Some may want their doctor to make all the decisions, simply clueing them into the "plan" as each new hurdle is faced. Other patients want to be involved with each step of decision making, want to be given choices and information, be educated on each diagnosis and treatment. Simply put, some people want a consistent, open dialogue with their doctor, while some simply want to trust in their healthcare professional and not get in his or her way.

In my opinion, it comes down to similar personalities being able to work together that makes for the best patient-doctor symbiosis. This is not a one-size-fits-all consideration, and surely, while reputations and referrals go a long way in giving you much-needed insights, ultimately the doctor you choose will depend on the personal criteria you want to see met.

In looking for the right oncologist (cancer doctor), do as much exploring across Google as you want about doctors, but be sure to let the clear light of practicality into your decisions as well. You may not live in a town that offers many options where cancer treatments are concerned. As your treatment progresses, you will likely feel a lot worse before you feel better, and traveling anywhere farther than a few miles from your home might be difficult or too exhausting . . . even if somebody else is doing the driving. Also, ask yourself how far you'd be willing and able to travel to seek out a second (or even a third) opinion; I'd always advise doing so, but it's simply not always possible for each patient to get around so easily.

My mom got lucky the first time she was diagnosed with cancer in that she found a doctor close to our home that she trusted, and he included her in every decision. She received all her treatments at his office. This is what she wanted in her doctor, and fortunately, this is what she got. Since I was a college kid at the time, I can only imagine how difficult I would have made her doctor visits, peppering her doctor with questions. If I had only known what I know now!

My mom was offered the option to go to a larger cancer center for a second opinion, even given the option of other treatment options, but she never wanted to travel far and was confident in the care she received from her cancer team. And they were wonderful, I must say. But you might not have so many choices where you live, or you might be presented with so many it makes your head spin.

We'll get into types of cancer in the next chapter, but another major consideration here is whether a doctor in your area specializes in treating the type of cancer you have. You may want to consider seeing a specialist for your initial consultation or second opinion before you decide if this is the doctor for you. Again, where this doctor is located—how near or how far—can factor into your decision making.

Consider simple, practical matters like: does your doctor have ample parking at his or her office? Does he or she have adequate access to public transportation if you happen to be making your visits without a car? What are this doctor's office hours? Is he/she affiliated with another doctor who might be able to see you when you can't travel to a certain location? Does this doctor take your insurance or have they been recommended by your health insurance company? All these issues are ones to consider.

I know there is a lot to think about, but again, these initial decisions are ones that will greatly come to factor into your care down the line.

When you finally settle on a facility or an oncologist to begin treatment, I advise approaching this potential doctor as if you are conducting an interview. I know we are supposed to hold these men and women up in our minds with some rarified regard, but if you don't ask the hard questions of them, who will? As LeAnn advised me in her matter-of-fact sassiness, "Hey, these doctors are working for you!"

You may be thinking, I don't even know what questions to ask, so how can I interview a doctor? Just take a breath and think about what you want from your cancer doctor, as much what you always wanted from a healthcare professional. Overall, it really should come down to the same goal: you finding someone you can communicate with.

As Phil says about this subject:

First and foremost, you want to be looking for a general point person on your healthcare team. This is the person who you can talk to freely and that communicates well with you. In the best of all possible worlds this will be your oncologist, but not always.

Depending on how big the team is, where it is you are going for treatment, and even the particular doctor or doctors involved, sometimes it might be a nurse practitioner who answers all your questions, is the person who, in the best-case scenario, becomes your friend through your cancer. In the case of a surgeon, for instance, where someone has a type of cancer that requires just surgery, you probably won't get the surgeon on the phone with you all that often. But the surgeon will likely have a point person who can answer your questions, who can explain things in layman's terms. It's like a coach on a team; they are usually not the person you talk to directly; they are too busy getting the plays in order, figuring who is playing what position; you probably will go to the assistant coach with the everyday questions.

Either way, you need to find someone who will communicate with you well, regularly, and keeps the jargon to a minimum.

This goes beyond the initial diagnosis and all those questions you will have about it, even beyond your treatment. There is a broader landscape to focus on here as this event unfolds in your life, more than just what kind of cancer you have and what the treatment will be. You are going to need someone to be there for you for a while. When things go wrong, as they will, or not even wrong precisely but when things get tough, like with side effects, etc., you are going to want someone who will be there through the long haul answering your questions and helping allay your fears. You don't want to be left just going round and round with your questions and concerns, like pushing a piece of spaghetti around on a plate.

I'm not treating patients anymore, but I came across someone recently who had a relative who I treated. We didn't realize at first that we had any connection. But when my name was mentioned, this family member said that the thing they most remembered about me was that I took the time to talk with their family member, the cancer patient, that I listened and then answered their questions. I always had the time to do that for them, and of course, while this is a wonderful compliment to me directly and I am happy to hear I impacted someone's life this way, it also illustrates what I do feel is most important, first and foremost. I have often heard that people go out to get a second opinion less because they don't feel they get adequate care but that they can't communicate with their doctor.

The above speaks to the person and healthcare professional I know Philip to be. He is one hundred percent accurate in his assessment of his best qualities, and I am not saying that only because he is my friend and a colleague I respect so much. And I couldn't agree more, that when you get that cancer diagnosis and start to put together your healthcare team, **you should be** as diligent as you can, or get your caregiver on the case, to make sure you hire that answer man/woman who you can trust to be with you for a very long time who communicates with you perfectly—right from the outset.

Ask your friends and loved ones what they want ***answered***. Quite often they will ask things you aren't thinking of, or their questions might prompt additional queries from you. If this list of uncertainties gets too long, write them down. In fact, write them down no matter how many questions you come up with. Buy a journal, or even scribble your questions in the margins of this book. I can't reiterate enough that although cancer has come into your life, it has not taken the control of your life away from you. This initial vetting of your doctor is the one area, and one of the first, where you definitely have a say. Do everything you can to make sure your concerns and queries are answered with every new healthcare professional you see.

For LeAnn's specific (and harrowing) set of circumstances, especially coming from a place where she had no knowledge of cancer, its diagnosis and treatment, and being the caregiver, she met the challenge of finding the best healthcare team for her son and adapting quickly to the challenges coming upon her family. As she says:

When somebody is diagnosed with cancer, from that date onward, your life changes forever. Suddenly your mind is swirling and you realize you don't know enough. Sixteen thousand children are diagnosed with cancer each year, and the population is even smaller than that when you consider kids who are diagnosed with brain cancer, which is what my son Cameron was diagnosed with (a malignant brain rumor called medulloblastoma), but what did we know about it?

Suddenly we were part of a very small club, certainly not one anyone ever wants to join, but one that is very supportive and welcoming all the same, and we had people contacting us.

But it was a constant battle to have Cameron's doctors explain the steps so we could educate ourselves. Your brain pretty quickly gets filled, it isn't easy to keep everything clear, and frankly it's your child lying there sick, so pretty much all bets are off where manners are concerned. I had to say to doctors all the time, I need you to explain things to me so I can sleep at night, best as I was sleeping. If you find a doctor refusing to do this, he or she might be the wrong doctor for you, it's as simple as that.

Do not accept the first answer if it doesn't make any sense to you. This is where I think patient advocacy can really come in.

Advocates can walk through the journey with you, provide a new set of ears; even your friends can help in his regard. I'd advise keeping a journal by your bed as well. Questions came to me all the time; taking a shower getting up in the middle of the night, I found that journal was an invaluable tool.

Generally, I found that the doctors and nurses who work in pediatric cancer are above and beyond wonderful. They have a truly unique view of things and they really love the kids. You hear of nurses shaving their heads in solidarity, so many instances that bring tears to your eyes proving how much these doctors, nurses, and the staff so love these kids. We found great people throughout Cameron's illness; it was just making sure we understood at all times what was happening.

⟡⟡⟡

If a doctor balks at a question or doesn't seem to want to take the time to walk you through the initial stages of your care, this should be a bright red flag to you that this professional might not be the best fit for you.

Here are some basic questions you should be asking your potential doctor:

- What types of cancer does this doctor treat?
- What hospital do they have privileges in?
- Will you be seeing him/her during treatment, or will other oncologists be managing your care also?
- What are this doctor's office hours?
- Who will care for you in the event the doctor is not available?
- What is the protocol for emergency situations?
- How can this doctor be contacted after hours?
- What medical insurance does this doctor's office accept?

After talking with the doctor, did you feel that she/he:

- Listened to your concerns and questions and was able to answer them
- Provided information about your disease and treatment options in a way that you could understand
- Had a helpful and compassionate staff
- Took their time and did not rush you (or by extension their staff did not rush you)
- Explained to you the resources that they have available, and who their team members are

Remember, not every cancer doctor has a winning bedside manner. Some men and women who care for us can only do so if they distance themselves fr om the emotion of caring for sick people and the possibility that some patients die. In my experience, some of the best doctors, people who I'd want at my side in every emergency, are simply not all that warm and fuzzy in their approach. Fantastically competent though they are, they simply don't know how to hold somebody's hand or talk softly. Phil shared with me that when he went to medical school, his college taught doctor-patient communication, but initially medical study was not set up to have doctors consider their bedside manner.

But if it is important to you to have a doctor with a warm personality, quite frankly, you need to look for one.

So, where do you start the search for a doctor? You may have been referred to an oncologist by your primary care doctor, or whatever doctor diagnosed your cancer. These referrals are important; don't take them lightly. Just remember, you can always feel free to look for other options. Here are a couple of possibilities to consider:

- If you weren't referred to an oncologist by your primary care doctor, does he/she have any recommendations? Why would he/she recommend a particular oncologist?

- Would your primary care doctor go to this oncologist for treatment? Send a family member to him/her?

- Is there a list of oncologists that participate in your health insurance plan?

- How far do you want to travel for your care? Would you prefer to stay close to home, or are you willing/able to travel to find a doctor?

- Do you have any friends/family members who have been treated by an oncologist? Would they recommend their doctor?

- Is there a facility near you that has a stellar reputation for cancer care? A place that you have either heard of or a loved one or friend might recommend?

You can find a whole bunch of sources online from which to vet cancer doctors, including cancer advocacy sites and even sites that allow people to grade their doctors (I list some in the Resources page of this chapter), but remember every patient may be expecting something different from their doctor, and not all of their "grades" may be relevant to your situation. The nice thing about patient advocacy group sites is that they often concern themselves with specific types of cancer and may highlight doctors that specialize in your type of cancer and treatment.

You should also find out from those doctors you visit if they are board certified in oncology and/or hematology. This means that they have undergone additional training specific to diagnosing and treating cancer and are required to take ongoing medical education so they are up to date on new research and treatments. Ask also what other additional or specialized training they might have regarding cancer and even other disciplines. For instance, the cancer doctor who has some background in nutrition above and beyond the normal courses taught in medical school might be able to help you with nausea during your treatment in ways you haven't considered. If you are a person who is especially interested in complementary cancer treatments (something I will get into in the treatment chapter), you might want to make sure the doctor(s) you are vetting are sympathetic to this approach to cancer care as much as you.

As Joyce weighs in:

Navigating real information online vs. not-so-good-legitimate sites, evaluating and choosing a treatment site; the path to finding the scenario that works for an individual/family is really what you're most after during these initial stages. You should make the most out of the academic or a community-based accredited cooperative sites, but I suggest also seeking information and resources and support from national or local cancer advocacy organizations.

Cancer advocacy organizations usually are focused on types of cancers and are there to provide live information by phone in addition to their website. These organizations have national or local patient information specialists that can be reached by phone. The people who answer the phone are there specifically to give callers information, to help build connections. These advocacy and support groups are invaluable. These are deep resources for so much of what a patient will face initially, as well as advising people to what they might come to expect down the line, from the normal sequence of diagnoses, as well as all the way down the line when someone is facing certain financial concerns. At lots of these sites, patients will be able to connect with other people's similar experiences, not just technical information, and this can help someone feel that they are not alone.

Ideally, a family should be able to feel they made the best choice at the time, with the best information available. One way to make sure you feel you're making the right decisions is to consider another opinion. Many people feel uncomfortable with that, as they feel their doctor may see it as a negative toward them. I often hear people say they like their doctor and they don't want them to feel they are unhappy by seeking a second opinion. It is OK to seek a second opinion to learn how another cancer team would evaluate and recommend care. Seeking a second opinion at a reputable cancer center, with clinical trials, is a good option to learn about the whole picture and options.

And she adds, reiterating what Phil and LeAnn say above:

Communication with healthcare providers is essential. Healthcare literacy is an issue in the general population, and in the scenario of a very stressful, serious, and complicated diagnosis, it can create miscommunication. Empowering a patient/family to ask questions, and to request that information be provided in a way they find meaningful is really important. Asking questions in several ways—asking for pictures, percentages, numbers, examples of other patients like themselves—are all good examples. Patients and their support should leave a consultation with an HCP feeling they understand the information provided and the decisions they are to make.

Learn of your potential doctor's history treating your cancer specifically as well as how long have they been practicing. Get a good overview of the doctor's professional history. It's OK to ask. Remember what LeAnn said: these people are working for you.

Now, let's consider the importance of not only the doctor, but where that doctor works. In lots of ways, the clinic the doctor practices in can reflect the doctor and how he/she practices. As Joyce adds: "Finding where to be treated can be a little tricky, as not everyone has adequate mobility or resources, but it's the 'critical thinking' part of the process here that is important. My experience is that this is the one area people most often feel compelled to charge into, with most simply finding a facility locally."

Your comfort with the facility is important. I know of some densely populated areas that have some of the biggest and brightest cancer care facilities in the country, but not everybody is comfortable going to these facilities. Maybe there isn't enough privacy in the treatment area and you'd rather have a quiet area to yourself, or maybe it's too private and you'd like to be around other patients that you can talk with while getting your treatment. Many of us feel comforted by a hospital or care center with a seemingly large reach across the community and country, and some may view a smaller practice as more personable. Some doctors and the places they work advertise that they are well-versed on the latest treatments and trials (you can check this easily to make sure if this is true), while others have great success at only one thing that they do best. What I am advising here is to vet your doctor, their staff, and the facility they work out of. Believe me, a receptionist who is lackadaisical about passing messages along won't be somebody you'll want to deal with later on.

I know there is a lot to consider: how to find a doctor; what to ask him or her when you do find them; considering the facility they work at. But remember, if you don't ask those initial questions and don't do even the most basic research, down the line it's going to be hard back-peddling as you wish for your doctor to suddenly act differently than they have all along. At these initial stages of choosing who will take care of you, you have every right to ask any question you like. The answers you get (or don't get) and the way you are answered will clue you in if this healthcare professional is right for you. There is no flaw in you if you fail to connect with someone or even a facility.

Last, I'd like to address a sticky subject that I brushed over at the beginning of this chapter . . . the second opinion. In my view, if your doctor downplays the idea or doesn't even want to discuss you going for a second opinion, you should consider strongly if this doctor is for you. I won't kid you, some doctors used to have an underlying concern that if they encouraged their patients to seek a second opinion that they might indeed be setting themselves up to lose that patient. In what I see these days in oncology, second opinions are often recommended, or even set up for you by your own doctor. Many doctors are affiliated with other (sometimes) bigger facilities—my mother's doctor was—and can get into quick consultations or readily recommend their patient to a colleague. Remember, seeking a second opinion is your right, and in fact, if you have the time and can manage the travel, I do highly recommend getting that second opinion.

Here is a quick reference for the type of doctors you could encounter during your cancer treatment:

Medical Oncologist: A doctor who is trained to diagnose and treat cancer. Medical oncologists may prescribe a variety of different treatments for your type of cancer, including chemotherapy, hormonal therapy, targeted therapy, or immunotherapy. Often, but not always, medical oncologists will be the coordinating doctor if you have a team of doctors involved in your care.

Hematologist: A doctor who is trained to diagnose and treat disorders of the blood, including cancers that start in the blood, such as leukemia. Hematologists may prescribe a variety of treatments for your type of cancer, including chemotherapy, targeted therapy, immunotherapy, or stem-cell transplant.

Radiation Oncologist: A doctor who is trained to treat cancer with ionizing radiation. Radiation oncologists will often coordinate with a medical oncologist to determine the appropriate treatment plan for each patient.

Surgical Oncologist: A doctor who is trained as a surgeon and who specializes in the surgical management of tumors.

Neuro-oncologist: A doctor with special training, often in both neurology and oncology, and who specializes in treating tumors of the brain and spinal cord.

Gynecologic Oncologist: A doctor who specializes in diagnosing and treating gynecologic cancers, such as ovarian, cervical, uterine, and endometrial. Gynecologic oncologists are trained as both surgeons and medical oncologists.

Pediatric Oncologist or Pediatric Hematologist: A doctor who specializes in treating children or teens who have been diagnosed with cancer. These physicians undergo advanced training to be able to evaluate and treat the unique nature of care in children.

Pathologist: A physician who examines tissues and lab tests and interprets the results in order to diagnose a patient's cancer.

There are some wonderful men and women out there working hard to cure patients with cancer. I hope you find the one who specifically fits your needs, but remember, it is up to you to be as proactive as you can in your searching. And don't forget to ask questions, lots of questions. The first way you take control of your health in this most dire of circumstances is to find the best doctor for you.

Takeaways

- Knowing that your doctor understands your type of cancer and feeling that they will communicate with you openly are critical factors to consider when you choose a doctor.
- Get a journal or a notebook that you can easily carry with you, to write down questions that you want to ask and the answers you get. The amount of information you are dealing with can be overwhelming and hard to keep track of.
- In considering your oncologist, you need to also consider the location of their clinic:
  ◊ How far is the facility from you?
  ◊ Do you feel comfortable there, and are they the best facility for the type of cancer you have?
  ◊ If you will be getting treatments in a facility, is it an environment that you are going to be comfortable in?
- Getting a second, and even a third, opinion is your right.

RESOURCES:

Certainly one of the most reliable sources for cancer information is the **American Cancer Society**, https://www.cancer.org/, 1-800-ACS-2345 (toll free).

Healthgrades' **National Health Index**, https://www.healthgrades.com/. Twenty-five U.S. cities exist in their network for connecting patients, healthcare providers, and hospitals.

U Compare Healthcare, http://www.ucomparehealthcare.com/, provides net-based tools for anyone looking to compare the various healthcare services available.

American Society of Clinical Oncology Cancer.Net, http://www.cancer. net, provides doctor-approved information for cancer patients, and offers suggestions on how to navigate your cancer diagnosis and care.

Chapter 3

What Type of Cancer Do I Have?

Finding out you have cancer can come in a variety of ways. Perhaps you found a lump and went to see your doctor, or something showed up during a routine checkup or screening. Visits for ordinary ailments can sometimes reveal unexpected causes. It could be that you started to bruise easily, because your blood didn't clot as it once did; or that you suddenly become more prone to fevers and infections. Maybe a family history of cancer made you start asking questions and undergo some tests. Or maybe you were feeling that something was just "not right."

As I mentioned previously, I went in for a routine dermatology checkup, questioning if a mole on my lower back was normal. From there it escalated . . . at least until I could calm myself, consider my options, and make a few phone calls.

I was extremely lucky. My melanoma was caught early, and I didn't need any further treatment. I had to go in for follow-up visits every three months for the next three years, and every appointment stressed me out. Was my cancer back? I worried every single time I sat in the exam room waiting for the doctor, and I'd come to have over fifteen biopsies over the next five years, some of which came back abnormal but none of them melanoma.

I'm now fifteen years past my diagnosis and I'm cancer free, yet every year I go in for a checkup, I worry that they will find more; I don't think the fear ever fully goes away. It's a recurring theme for anyone who has survived any kind of cancer and, I'm sorry to say, not something you ever get over worrying about. Even if you are lucky enough to pass that all-important five-year mark cancer free and your doctor changes the plan to a once-a-year screening, you can still feel like you are never totally free of it. Screening can raise stressful echoes of your cancer and how it blew through your life and remind you that it could, for seemingly no reason at all, reappear.

Just remember, finding cancer early on greatly improves the outcome, and screening is simply looking for a problem to nip it in the bud.

This vigilance is smart.

Being screened is your best bet to find cancer early.

Screening/Scans

From a cancer screening perspective, many tests are currently used; screening is the broader term, and would include things like mammograms, colonoscopies, etc. The idea behind screening is to catch cancer early and make treatment less invasive and more effective. There is a risk for potential overdiagnosis (picking up cancers that might never do any harm) or false-positive results, which can add significant stress to patients while they wait for confirmatory testing. It all comes down to weighing the risks. I've had abnormal mammograms that have required further testing and even biopsy, and it certainly adds stress, but I would rather do whatever I can to find something early. If one of my sons had something show up in a blood test and needed a scan or screening, I wouldn't hesitate for a second making sure he went for whatever was suggested to test him further. God knows how many people have found cancer and found it early enough to save their lives through screenings and scans.

Genetic testing is also being done more often as we begin to understand the connection between genetics and our risk of developing cancer. But this is usually only recommended for patients who have a family history of cancer. Even then, meeting with a genetic counselor is critical to understand what it all means.

As I work in this field and come to understand ever more about cancer and its treatments, I realize I am armed against cancer in a way few people are. As I tried to do in the previous chapter, giving you what I feel was good advice about seeking out your doctor, here I want to answer your questions about the cancer you have. (In the next chapter I will get into treatment.)

Understanding Your Diagnosis

According to the National Cancer Institute (NCI), there are over one hundred types of cancer, and they are classified based on the organ or tissue they started in. However, many cancers have unique attributes that can further differentiate them from this general type. For example, breast cancer is one of the one hundred types identified by the NCI. However, within breast cancer are different subtypes, like ductal or lobular, depending on which specific cells the cancer started in. The process of defining the type of cancer you have and what will happen for your future treatments can be daunting. Before we talk types, though, let's talk about what cancer is exactly.

In simple terms, cancer is abnormal cells dividing and growing out of control. Something has affected the genetic material in these cells, and they begin to crowd or "kill off" normal cells. While not all causes of cancer are known, research has shown that some factors can change or damage DNA, leading to cancer. Certain factors are ones I'm sure you are aware of: exposure to certain chemicals or substances, tobacco use, and too much exposure to ultraviolet light. A person can also be at higher risk of developing certain types of cancer because of inherited genes.

How do your doctors know that you have cancer? They may have conducted several tests or may be scheduling additional ones soon to gather more information and confirm the diagnosis.

In addition to the screening procedures that are used to help detect cancer, more detailed tests are used to diagnose and stage cancer. These include biopsies; imaging tests such as PET, CT, MRI; as well as laboratory tests.

Biopsies involve removing tissue so it can be examined to determine the presence or extent of disease. Biopsies can be obtained in several different ways depending on where the abnormal area is found.

Bone Marrow Biopsy: A sample of bone marrow is drawn out of the back of your hipbone using a long needle. Bone marrow biopsies are used to diagnose blood cancers such as leukemia, lymphoma, and multiple myeloma. You will likely receive medicine to numb the area and minimize your discomfort.

Endoscopic Biopsy: A thin, flexible tube with a light on the end is inserted into your body, through your mouth, rectum, urinary tract, or a small incision in your skin, in order to collect tissue. Where the tube is inserted depends on the location of the suspicious area. You may receive a sedative or anesthetic before the procedure.

Needle Biopsy: A special needle is used to extract tissue. This type of biopsy is primarily used on tumors that your doctor can feel through your skin. You will receive medicine to numb the area being biopsied to minimize the pain.

Surgical Biopsy: Surgery may be required to reach the suspicious area and to collect tissue. Depending on where the tumor is, a surgeon may remove the entire tumor and some surrounding normal tissue for testing, or may remove part of the tumor.

Imaging tests are also used for diagnosis and staging (although they may be used for screening as well, like MRI, which is used in addition to mammograms for women at high risk for developing breast cancer).

Positron Emission Tomography (PET) Scan: An imaging test that uses a radioactive substance, called a tracer, to look for disease in the body. The tracer is injected into the patient's vein prior to the scan and is absorbed by the body's tissues and organs. When the scan is performed, doctors can see if certain areas are highlighted and determine where cancer is present in a person's body.

Computed Tomography (CT) Scan: An X-ray procedure that combines many images with the help of a computer, allowing radiologists to see cross-sectional views and three-dimensional images of internal organs and structures within the body.

Magnetic Resonance Imaging (MRI): A test that uses a magnetic field and pulses of radio wave energy to make pictures of organs and structures within the body.

Laboratory tests, such as blood or urine tests, may also be used to help diagnose cancer, although they are currently not able to do so on their own. Blood samples can also be used to determine if you have any genetic markers that are important to your diagnosis and treatment options.

In the case of a biopsy, once tissue is collected, it is sent to a pathologist, who looks at cells from the tumor (or blood or bone marrow) to document changes. The pathologist will determine what type of cells the cancer originated from (and therefore where it started) and how closely the tumor cells still resemble normal tissue cells. Remember that **the type of cancer you have is based upon where it began**, its original tissue or cell type.

This determination is exceedingly important, as the oncologist will base your treatment on the initial cancer you present; different treatments are employed for different kinds of cancers.

In addition to aiding with an initial diagnosis, imaging tests are also used to help determine if the cancer has spread beyond the tumor site, to nearby lymph nodes or other areas of the body. When cancer spreads, patients are sometimes confused and say things like: "Well, I have breast cancer, but I also now have cancer in my lymph nodes, and then . . ." This is usually all the same cancer. In rare cases, it could be separate cancers. If you have any doubt or confusion, ask your doctor to clarify for you. My mother started with breast cancer, but later when her cancer came back, it would begin again in her breast then eventually metastasize to her rib cage, her shoulder, liver, and brain. But from the first time cancer was found in her, to the second, then the third, when it would eventually take her life, it was all breast cancer.

Once all information is gathered, a report will be sent to a doctor specializing in cancer—*an oncologist or hematologist*—which they will use to determine appropriate treatment. **You should get a copy of this report for your records.** You may not understand everything in it, but it may be helpful having it in your possession later on.

Time and again here I will make the point that **having information is critical to your care**.

How Bad Is My Cancer?

Your doctor will examine all the information available, from all the tests that have been done, and identify what type and stage of cancer you have. Cancer is usually classified as "solid tumor" (starting in the tissue/bones) or "liquid tumors"/"hematologic cancers" (which are leukemia, lymphoma, and multiple myeloma). Leukemia starts in the blood cells and bone marrow, lymphoma starts in the lymphatic system, and multiple myeloma, also starting in the blood/bone marrow, is cancerous plasma cells.

The stage describes how your cancer has affected your body and how advanced it is. For solid tumors (those that don't start in the blood-forming tissue or the patient's immune system), doctors will use what is called the **TNM** staging system. This is based on the size of your tumor (**T**), whether or not the cancer has spread to your lymph nodes (**N**), and whether or not the cancer has spread farther in your body or metastasized (**M**). Lower numbers (stages I and II) are used for cancer that is found earlier, and higher numbers (stages III and IV) indicate that your cancer is more advanced.

For other types of cancer, such as leukemia, lymphoma, and multiple myeloma, TNM staging does not work. The following systems are used for these cancers:

Leukemia

For leukemia, doctors will look at the number of cancer cells, as well as what type of cells they are, to identify which type and subtype of leukemia you have; *acute* (cancer progressing quickly) vs. *chronic* (a cancer not progressing quickly); and *lymphocytic* (cancer starting in the lymphoid stem cells) vs. *myelogenous* (cancer starting in the myeloid stem cells).

Lymphoma

Lymphoma is divided into two categories, *Hodgkin's lymphoma (HL)* and *non-Hodgkin's lymphoma (NHL)*. While both types start in the lymphocytes, if a specific type of abnormal cell called a Reed-Sternberg cell is detected, then the lymphoma is classified as Hodgkin's lymphoma.

- Hodgkin's lymphoma is staged (the determination of how far it has progressed) using what is called the Lugano system. Hodgkin's lymphoma generally starts in the lymph nodes. If it spreads, it is usually to another set of nearby lymph nodes. It has four stages, labeled I, II, III, and IV, depending on the number and location of lymph node areas affected.

- Non-Hodgkin's lymphoma is staged using what is called the Ann Arbor staging system. Roman numerals I–IV are used to show how extensive the disease is in the lymph nodes. If the cancer has also affected the spleen, an "S" will be added after the Roman numeral, and if it has affected an organ outside of your lymph system, an "E" will be added after the numeral.

I know I'm giving you a lot of information, and for the most part, these specifics will probably pass you by as you weigh other concerns. But there just might come a time when you'll want to manage a deep dive through all the reports you have been given to truly understand all that is going on. I want to provide you with as much ammunition to fight what you are going through.

Types

Finally, we come to more specific information on types of cancer. In addition to considering the organ or location where your cancer started, cancer is also classified by the type of cell that formed it. These types include:

Sarcoma: A malignant tumor that begins growing in connective tissues such as muscle, bone, fat, or cartilage.

Carcinoma: A malignant tumor that starts in the surface layer of an organ or body part and may spread to other parts of the body.

Leukemia: A type of cancer that starts in tissue that forms blood, such as the bone marrow. It causes abnormal blood cells to be produced, displacing normal blood. This can lead to infection, shortage of red blood cells, bleeding, and other complications.

Multiple Myeloma: A type of cancer that affects the plasma cells in blood, leading to damage to bones, immune system, kidneys, and red blood cells.

Lymphoma:A malignant tumor originating in the immune system cells, such as lymph nodes.

Melanoma: Cancer that begins in cells that become melanocytes, which are specialized cells that make melanin, or the pigment that gives skin and moles their color.

Central Nervous System cancers: A type of cancer that begins in tissues such as the brain or spinal cord.

Questions to Ask Your Doctor

Here are some examples of questions you may have for your doctor directly related to your cancer. There will certainly be many other questions that come up as you learn more about your disease, your treatment options, and the impact that cancer is having on your life. As I did in the previous chapter, I urge you to write these questions down and keep track of the answers you are given. Generally, what you want to know initially is:

~ What type of cancer do I have?
~ Where exactly is it located?
~ What is the stage of my cancer and what does this mean for my immediate health and treatment options?
~ Has my cancer spread to my lymph nodes or anywhere else?
~ How is staging used to determine my cancer treatment?
~ What is my chance of recovery?
~ What are the risk factors for this disease? Is there something in my environment or lifestyle that I should be changing to help myself,

for example, exposure to chemicals, smoke, etc. Is there a risk to other family members?

~ Is this type of cancer caused by genetic factors? Are other members of my family at risk?

~ How many people are diagnosed with this type of cancer each year?

~ Where can I find more information about my cancer?

~ Should I get a second opinion?

My Diagnosis

~ Based on the tests that have been done, and what I've learned from my doctors, I understand that I have _____ cancer, and that it is considered _____stage.

I hate to whittle all these concerns down to the simple paragraph above. But these are the basic facts when it comes to your cancer . . . ***what type is it*** and ***what stage is it in***? As we will come to see, your treatment options are determined from the answers to these two basic questions. As I mentioned before and will touch on again, it is your right to search out another opinion about the cancer you have and what can be done about it. But first and foremost, you need to know what you are specifically up against with this invader in your body and what stage it is at.

Takeaways

• Find out what kind of cancer you have. Find out where it started in your body and, if it has spread, where it is now. This information will determine your treatment options.

- Ask if there are other types of tests that will be done to give your doctor more details.
- Research, and question all you can about the kind of cancer you have.

RESOURCES:

The **American Cancer Society,** https://www.cancer.org/, 1-800-ACS-2345 (toll free). The ACS's website has resources and research for all types of cancer, diagnosis, treatment options . . . and so much more.

The **National Breast and Cervical Cancer Early Detection Program** (NBCCEDP), https://www.cdc.gov/cancer/nbccedp/index.htm, helps low-income and uninsured women to find and facilitate breast and cervical cancer screenings.

The **National Cancer Institute** (NHI), https://www.cancer.gov/, proclaims it is "the nation's leader in cancer research." It provides a deep well of information.

Cancer Treatment Centers of America (CTCA), https://www.cancercenter.com/, 855-412-1358, constantly updates blog posts, research on treatment and cancer types, and so many other concerns for patients and caregiver.

The **Leukemia and Lymphoma Society,** www.lls.org, 1-800-955-4572. For patients with leukemia, lymphoma, or myeloma, the LLS offers assistance on services and treatments, transportation to treatment centers, and financial assistance for insurance co-payments. They have chapters in all fifty states.

The **Cancer Support Community,** https://www.cancersupportcommunity.org/, 888-793-9355 (toll free). Like the AMS, the CSC offers a multi–web page resource for the many questions you might have about cancer and where to find support.

The **National Cancer Institutes'** Seer Training Modules, https://training.seer.cancer.gov, are an invaluable resource of web pages about all aspects of cancer.

The **National Comprehensive Cancer Network,** https://www.nccn.org/, is another invaluable resource for fighting cancer.

American Society of Clinical Oncology Cancer.Net, http://www.cancer. net, provides doctor-approved information for cancer patients, and offers suggestions on how to navigate your cancer diagnosis and care.

Counseling & Emotional Support

The **Cancer Care Organization**, https://www.cancercare.org/, 1-800-813-HOPE, offers face-to-face, online, and telephone counseling for a multitude of concerns.

The **American Psychosocial Oncology Society**, https://apos-society.org/, 1-866-276-7443 offers telephone referrals for counseling.

Cancer Information and Counseling Line, http://amc.org.s104393. gridserver.com/programs.html, 1-800-525-3777, an affiliate of AMC Cancer Research Center, offers telephone counseling to cancer patients and their families.

Chapter 4

Treatment

For most people, a cancer diagnosis equates to getting chemotherapy, being nauseous, losing their hair, and possibly dying. My hope in writing this book is to give you ammunition, power, and a chance to take control of your life when you have been diagnosed with cancer. Although I can't be there sitting next to you as you go through one of the scariest times of your life, the good news is that you don't have to feel alone. And the better news is that we are getting smarter every day in regards to our understanding of cancer, how best to treat it, and how to minimize the side effects of treatment. I'm not saying you might not lose your hair or that you will feel great during treatment, but the medical community has made great progress in the last twenty years to find the right treatment for specific types of cancer and to find ways to prevent or treat the side effects.

The type of treatment your oncologist will suggest depends on many factors: the type of cancer you have, where it's located, how large it is, and if it has spread. The goal of treatment is to remove as many cancer cells from your body as possible so that your cancer goes into remission (meaning that the signs and symptoms of your cancer are reduced), or to prolong your life as long as possible. Remission can be partial or complete. In a complete remission, all signs and symptoms of cancer have disappeared. If you remain in complete remission for five years or more, some doctors may say that you are cured. By the time your doctor starts discussing treatment, you will likely feel overwhelmed with all the information. I'll try and offer some help by presenting and explaining some of the most common treatment options and a broad overview of what to expect from each. As you can imagine, treatments can affect everyone differently, from their effectiveness to their side effects.

Surgery

If your cancer has not spread and is in an area of your body where it can be removed, then surgery is often one of the primary treatments a surgeon or an oncologist will suggest. The goal is to remove the entire tumor, reducing the risk of it growing back or having it spread. Surgery can also be used to reduce the size of your tumor or remove tumors that may be causing you pain or other symptoms. As I told you, I was exceedingly lucky with my melanoma; after it was removed by my plastic surgeon, I did not have a recurrence. Quite often, though, a cancerous tumor can't simply be plucked from one's body.

Patient recovery time from surgery can differ, depending on the location of the tumor or tumors, how big they are, and the patient's general health. Luckily, today surgery is typically less invasive than it used to be, so postoperative recovery and pain can be shorter and more easily managed. This can be very important, as cancer patients sometimes heal more slowly because of the disease itself and the strain or disruptions it's causing in your body. Still, there are side effects from surgery for cancer (as there always are with any surgery). These can include:

- Pain, especially in the area where a tumor or tumors are taken. How much tissue is removed, how large your incision is, and generally where your surgery was will also affect your pain levels.

- <u>Fatigue</u>. Surgery is a shock to the body; your system will need time to recover from it, as well as from the anesthesia you are given. This fatigue comes from taxing your physical and mental resources.

- <u>Swelling</u>, <u>drainage</u>, <u>irritation</u>, and <u>numbness</u> at the localized area where the surgery occurred. The surgeon is cutting into your body, after all. It should come as no surprise that there are often physical complications from this.

- <u>The possibility of infection.</u> Again, your body has been cut into, and while your surgeon and his team are sure to be vigilant against the possibility of infection, complications can still occur. This is why it is imperative you change dressings at home as you are instructed and make sure to come in for doctor's visits as they are scheduled.

Surgery is often used in conjunction with another treatment, such as:

Chemotherapy

Chemotherapy ("chemo" to the layman) is the use of drugs to kill cancer cells. These drugs can travel throughout your body, through your blood, and reach almost all areas of your body (though some areas, such as the brain, can be difficult to get to because of what's called the blood-brain barrier, which can prevent many drugs from crossing over). Chemotherapy works by killing cells that are dividing rapidly, which cancer cells do. In my mother's case, a tumor was removed, but subsequent chemo treatments were prescribed to get the remaining cancer that was still in her body. Healthy cells that are growing and dividing are also damaged with the introduction of chemotherapy. This leads to many of the side effects you've heard that people suffer with this type of treatment. Healthy cells that are often affected by chemotherapy include:

- <u>Hair</u>. Many cancer patients suffer from their hair falling out while undergoing chemo. As I mentioned, my mom's hair did fall out initially, but it did grow back.

- <u>Bone marrow</u> (which is constantly producing blood cells). White blood cells can be depleted by chemotherapy, making patients more prone to infection. In some cases, red blood cell growth is compromised as well, which can cause some patients to become anemic and feel more tired. Platelet production can also be compromised with chemotherapy, and in some patients, this causes the person to be more prone to bruising and bleeding.

- <u>Digestive system</u>. Many patients find chemotherapy running riot on their digestive system; terrible nausea ensues. Diarrhea can also be an effect of chemotherapy. My mom's nausea was a problem through her earlier treatments but was more manageable during her later treatments, when newer anti-nausea drugs were available.

- In some cases, patients complain of <u>irritation to the skin</u> or suffer from <u>inflammation</u> like canker sores.

- <u>Fatigue</u>. This can result from anemia that might occur, as chemotherapy often lowers red blood cell production.

The good news is that normal cells can replace or repair healthy cells that are adversely affected by chemotherapy. The damage to healthy cells doesn't usually last, and most side effects disappear once your treatment is over. Your doctor may give you other medicines during this kind of treatment to help alleviate some of the side effects you experience, such as medicine for nausea or to help shore up low blood counts. Complementary treatments can also help with these side effects. In just the past few years, many new drugs have been developed that help with the side effects of chemo.

Chemotherapy may be given as an oral medication (pill or capsule) or through an injection (intravenously, or IV) directly into your bloodstream. Some types of IV chemotherapy take a relatively short time to be administered, and you may get treated in a clinic, while others take a longer time and you may have to be admitted to the hospital to receive them.

Chemotherapy is administered on a regular schedule, called a "cycle," such as every three or four weeks. If you experience serious side effects, you may require changes, either to the amount you are receiving or to how often you are getting your treatment.

In some cases, chemotherapy alone may be able to cure your cancer, but often it is given in combination with other treatments, such as surgery and/or radiation, or radiotherapy. In the first of my mother's chemo treatments, her doctors would come to change her cocktail (they call it a cocktail simply because it is a mixture of more than one drug) because she had a severe reaction.

Radiotherapy/Radiation Therapy

Surgery is considered a *local* treatment; the tumor or tumors are *localized* in one area, and a surgeon goes in to get them. Chemo is not a localized treatment; a patient's entire system is assaulted by the chemo drugs; these drugs kill the cancer but also attack the entire body's system at the same time. Radiotherapy or radiation therapy can be a localized or regional treatment depending on how it is administered. In some cases, radioactive material can be inserted into the body in the location of the tumor, where it is needed to treat a small area. This approach can also minimize some side effects. Radiotherapy can also be administered from outside the body, *external radiotherapy*, via various types of machines. External radiotherapy can be used after surgery to treat surrounding areas, such as lymph nodes, that are in the region of where the tumor was. It can also be used without surgery to shrink tumors that can't be removed and to reduce symptoms. My mom received radiation therapy to her chest wall and lymph nodes after surgery to reduce the chances of the cancer coming back in the same area. She also received it later, directly to her brain, to reduce the size of her tumors when her cancer metastasized.

Prostate cancer happens to be one of the more common cancers where a radioactive material, "radioactive seeds," is inserted (brachytherapy); radioactive material is inserted to focus treatment and not affect other areas. The length of a course of radiotherapy treatment depends on the size and type of cancer being treated and where it is in the body. The patient might undergo one day of treatment or be treated over a few days or even weeks.

There are various forms of radiotherapy an oncologist might suggest. Some patients receive radiotherapy only to relieve symptoms, for example to reduce pain; this is called *palliative treatment.*

There is also a more extensive form of radiotherapy, *total body irradiation (TBI)*, quite like chemotherapy in that it affects the whole body and is used to kill bone marrow for patients with leukemia or lymphoma before they undergo a bone marrow transplant or stem cells are introduced into their system. Often combined with chemotherapy, this treatment destroys a patient's existing (and presumably diseased) bone marrow so that bone marrow or stem cells from the patient or their bone marrow donor can be reintroduced.

As with all the treatments illustrated above, radiotherapy affects people in different ways, so it's difficult to predict exactly how a specific patient will react to it until they undergo the treatment. Some people have only mild side effects, but for others, the side effects can be more severe.

Some general side effects of radiotherapy can include:

- <u>Fatigue</u>. Most people feel tired while they undergo radiotherapy, particularly if they are having treatment over several weeks. This is because the body is repairing the damage to healthy cells. Tiredness can also be the result of low levels of red blood cells (anemia).

- <u>Sore skin</u>. In the area of the body that's being treated, your skin may look reddened or darker than usual. It may also get dry and itchy. The skin may break, or small blisters can start to form in the area. The staff in the radiotherapy department can advise you on the best way of coping with this.

- <u>Hair falls out in the treatment area</u>. Hair in other parts of the body is not affected, though, and the hair over that specific treated area of your body that did fall out should begin to grow back again a few weeks after the treatment ends.

Like chemotherapy, radiation therapy is often combined with other treatments, such as surgery, chemotherapy, hormonal therapy, or biological therapy.

Hormone Therapy

Some cancers use hormones like fuel to grow or develop. When medicines are introduced into a patient's system to block or lower the amount of hormones in the body, cancer can no longer feed on those hormones. Of course, hormone therapy does not work for all cancers, but the cancers that often are hormone sensitive include breast cancer, prostate cancer, ovarian cancer, uterine, or endometrial cancer.

The side effects of hormone therapy are often worse at the start of the treatment; they usually settle down after a few weeks or months. They can include:

- Hot flashes and sweating
- Impotence
- Breast tenderness
- Weight gain
- Memory problems
- Mood swings
- Osteoporosis

Hormone therapy is often combined with other treatments, like surgery, where no chemo or radiotherapy is needed. In my mother's later treatments, she was given a form of hormone therapy. Hormonal therapy can cause complications for women hoping to have children later in life, as it can induce menopause and reduce fertility.

Biological Therapy

Biological therapy treatment is at the forefront of our present scientific knowledge. It is amazing stuff—almost science fiction, really—in that no drugs or chemicals are used. Instead, organic/biological material is grown in a lab (in great big vats), and this is introduced into the cancer patient to fight his or her cancer. These therapies are treatments that act on the actual processes in individual cells. They may:

- Stop cancer cells from dividing and growing
- Seek out cancer cells and kill them
- Encourage the immune system to attack cancer cells

Biological therapy is artificially produced antibodies that are made to target specific proteins on cells (cancer cells in this case), called antigens. These antibodies circulate throughout your body until they find and attach to the antigen, causing your immune system to destroy the cells that have the antigen.

Types of biological therapies:

- Targeted Therapies: antibodies (also referred to as monoclonal antibodies, or mAbs) work by recognizing and finding specific proteins on cancer cells. Each monoclonal antibody recognizes one particular protein and works in different ways depending on the protein they are targeting. So different monoclonal antibodies have to be made to target different types of cancer.

- Immunotherapy: Some therapies can trigger the immune system to attack and kill cancer cells. Although cancer cells are abnormal, they develop from normal cells, so they can be difficult for the immune system to spot. Some monoclonal antibodies simply attach themselves to cancer cells, making them easier for the cells of the immune system to find them. In addition to monoclonal antibodies, another promising biologic approach to immunotherapy is CAR (chimeric antigen receptor) T-cell therapy, where immune cells called T cells (a type of white blood cell) from a patient are changed in the lab so they can find and destroy cancer cells.

- Checkpoint Inhibitors: The immune system uses particular molecules to keep it from being overactivated and damaging healthy cells. These are known as checkpoints. Normally, T cells within your body's immune system would attack cancer cells. Some cancer cells make high levels of checkpoint molecules and switch off your immune system's response. Biological therapies that block checkpoint molecules are called checkpoint inhibitors.

- <u>Cancer Growth Blockers</u>: Cancer cells often make large numbers of molecules called growth factor receptors. These sit on the cell surface and send signals to help the cell survive and divide. Some monoclonal antibodies stop growth factor receptors from working properly, either by blocking the signal or the receptor itself. Once blocked, the cancer cell no longer receives the signals it needs to survive and multiply.
- <u>Conjugated Monoclonal Antibodies or Antibody-Drug Conjugates (ADC)</u>: Some monoclonal antibodies have drugs or radioactive substances attached to them. The mAbs finds the cancer cells and delivers the drug or radioactive substance directly to them.

The patient is given biological treatment as an injection under the skin (subcutaneous injection) or through a drip (infusion) into a vein. For some drugs, you have your first treatment into a vein, then further treatments as an injection under your skin. How often you have treatment and how many treatments you need will depend on your current state of health and the progression of your cancer.

Here again is another form of treatment my mother received during the third and last time she presented with cancer. She underwent a clinical trial and received a targeted therapy monoclonal antibody. It's a sad fact of recurring cancer diagnosis and the treatments that might follow: **a patient might undergo many different treatments in their lifetime as their doctor tries to save their life.**

Biological treatments can be more targeted than others, providing a better chance of treatment effectiveness. But there can still be serious side effects from these treatments; in some cases the patient's immune system is kicked into high gear by the introduction of the therapy, and doing so sometimes increases a person's chance for flu-like symptoms like chills, fever, and achiness. Sometimes this kind of treatment affects certain organs specifically or can increase a person's likelihood for allergic reactions or other type of hypersensitiveness.

Stem Cell Transplant or Bone Marrow Transplant

A stem cell transplant is used in some types of liquid tumor cancers such as leukemia, lymphoma, and myeloma; this kind of treatment can also be called **peripheral blood stem cell transplant (PBSCT) or bone marrow transplant**. Like biological therapies, peripheral blood stem cell transplantation is relatively new in medical science, whereas bone marrow transplantation has been used for years. The distinction between the terms "bone marrow" and "stem cell" comes from the source of the transplanted matter. If stem cells are taken from bone marrow and transplanted into a patient, this is called a bone marrow transplant; if the cells come from the bloodstream, this is known as a blood stem cell transplant.

For patients whose cancer is in their bone marrow and blood (like leukemia), the goal for treatment is to eradicate the cancer cells using high doses of chemotherapy or even whole-body radiotherapy, which kills all the cells—both good and bad—in their bone marrow, and then give the patient healthy stem cells so their body can begin to produce normal, healthy blood cells. Doctors may collect stem cells from the patient (called autologous transplant) or a matched donor (called allogeneic transplant) before treatment, and after a particularly high dose treatment of chemo or the like, this patient can have stem cells injected into a vein through a drip to replace those that the cancer treatment has killed.

These days, you're more likely to have a peripheral blood stem cell transplant than a bone marrow transplant. This is because your blood cell counts tend to recover faster via stem cell treatment; plus it's easier to collect stem cells from the blood than the bone marrow.

A patient can also receive a bone marrow transplant using bone marrow from a donor. This ***allogeneic transplant*** needs cells as similar as possible to the patient's; the cells can be from a brother or sister (what's called a "sibling match") or even someone not related to you but whose stem cells are similar to yours (a "matched unrelated donor").

Your doctor considers many different factors when deciding which type of transplant is right for you. At this stage, you will be presented with the best options for your particular case, and this is where the muscles you grew in chapter 2 should come into play, where you: ***ask questions***. There's a lot to find out here, and even if you have to go into your doctor's office with a journal and a whole bunch of questions, remember ultimately, you are in charge! You want to be especially knowledgeable about the transplant process, as you might require a donor for the cells you need. If you enlist another person into your treatment, in this very specific personal way, they deserve as much information as you can give them.

Regardless of the type of stem cell transplant you undergo, doctors will monitor and wait for your new cells to "engraft" (that's a word you will hear often if you undergo this treatment; it merely means waiting for the stem cells to "take" in the patient's system). The plan is that these new cells will begin to multiply and create new blood cells in your system. As with everything else, the time it takes for stem cells to engraft differs from individual to individual, typically taking anywhere from two to six weeks before your blood counts will begin to show that new cells are being produced.

The side effects of stem cell treatment can be numerous, and can be lessened or increased by a patient's overall health, what type (if any) of chemotherapy was used prior to the transplant, if radiation therapy was used prior to the transplant, and of course, the kind of transplant a person undergoes. Whether the cells transplanted were the patient's own or from a donor, and how close the donor match was will affect engrafting. The side effects here can include some we have seen before: nausea, temporary hair loss, but specific to stem cell or bone marrow transplants, some of the side effects you could experience are:

- Graft Versus Host Disease (GvHD). This is the main concern with allogeneic transplants. The white blood cells present within the transplanted tissue from the donor may attack the recipient's body's cells, which leads to GvHD. Patients might be prescribed immune-suppressing drugs to calm the battle their body wants to engage in over the transplant. Sometimes removal of a donor's T cells prior to transplantation (T cells are a white blood cell that helps control immune responses) can help prevent or reduce the impact of GvHD.

- Infection (bacterial, the most common). One of the frequent problems here; the transplant patient's white blood cells are at an all-time low, therefore their immune system is weakened. Allogeneic transplant patients have an even higher risk of infection because of the immune-suppressing drugs they may be receiving to prevent graft-versus-host disease, or GvHD.

- Bleeding & Anemia. Again, the result of compromised cells; low platelet count reduces a person's ability to clot properly, and a patient's red blood cell count lowers.

No matter the source of the stem cells or bone marrow, implantation is a complex process. Doctors monitor stem cell and bone marrow transplant patients quite proactively, as much to monitor engrafting as for possible side effects. This is truly cutting-edge treatment technology that is getting better every day.

Alternative vs. Complementary Therapies

The complaint I hear from doctors and healthcare works over any other these days is that too many of their patients are searching the Internet. In their fear or curiosity over an ache, pain, or cough, people naturally turn to the largest and most searchable listing of potential ailments known to man . . . the Internet. Doctors are besieged with men and women self-diagnosing. It's all they can do to assure their patients that they do not have what they fear they have.

Then there is the litany of TV ads we all see nightly offering to cure us of diseases we didn't even know existed. Drugs, whose possible side effects sound a lot worse than any disease they supposedly cure, are constantly advertised. You couldn't even begin to count how many doctors are asked to write prescriptions for all these meds daily.

My point being, we expect doctors to do the right thing and shield us from doing things that may be silly or dangerous out of our own fear and ignorance.

Then there are the hundreds of books, video interviews, blogs, and stories from folks supposedly cured by hundreds upon hundreds of natural medicines and methods, some supposedly tested, others simply rumored to be good. Some are even celebrity endorsed. As a general rule, if you have occasion to spin your mouse across the many sites out there, be aware that credible websites tend to end with a ".gov" or an ".org." Of course, you can find plenty of good information on sites ending with the normal

".com," it's just that these are usually places looking to make money, in some way, from their web pages.

I know full well that, as cancer patients, we are always looking for hope; it's no surprise that anyone with a life-threatening disease would consider anything to save their life. There are plenty of companies that want to legitimately provide people with that hope, and conversely, plenty that exploit a patient's need for it. Faced with our mortality, as we run through those classic psychological steps of denial, anger, bargaining, depression, and acceptance, often before the last step of acceptance we might try many different—see, *alternative*—measures for a cure, or even a little relief.

First and foremost, I think it is of the utmost importance to make the distinction between **complementary therapy** and **alternative therapy**. Though these phrases do not mean the same thing and they cover widely different treatments (and a world of difference between possible health concerns), I have often seen them combined into one phrase: complementary and alternative therapies (CAMs). While for the layman I know it is not always so easy to determine whether something is a complementary or an alternative therapy, there is an important distinction between the two, a difference that could greatly affect your health.

Complementary therapies are used alongside conventional medical treatments prescribed by your doctor. They can help people with cancer **to feel better** and may improve one's quality of life. They may also help you to better cope with symptoms caused by your cancer or the side effects that can come from the various treatments you undergo. A reputable complementary therapist won't claim that the therapy they introduce will cure your cancer, and they will always encourage you to discuss any therapies with your cancer doctor or GP.

Complementary therapies are available from many different types of people and organizations. These therapies include:

- Nutritional
- Aromatherapy
- Acupuncture
- Herbal Medicine
- Massage Therapy
- Visualization
- Yoga

Many health professionals are supportive of people with cancer using complementary therapies. Time and again they have seen reputable hard evidence that these therapies have helped their patients cope better with cancer and its various treatment side effects. But other health professionals have been and continue to be reluctant for their patients to use complementary therapies. This is because, while some of these therapies have been scientifically tested, many others have not, at least not in the same way as conventional treatments get tested. And despite the fact that yoga, herbal medicines, and acupuncture are considered natural, if and when we engage in any activity or begin to supplement our diets even with substances grown in our soil, these new therapies could interact negatively with more traditional cancer treatments.

Generally speaking, doctors need more studies to help them develop their knowledge about the best way to use complementary therapies and even explore ones that have not been fully developed.

Alternative therapies are used **instead of conventional medical treatment**. Some people may choose to use an alternative therapy instead of starting conventional cancer treatment, while others might stop conventional cancer treatment altogether and switch to an alternative therapy. But be cautioned here: while alternative therapists may claim to be able to cure your cancer with their treatments, so far *no scientific or medical evidence has shown that alternative therapies can cure cancer.*

This warning is worth repeating: *no scientific or medical evidence has shown that alternative therapies can cure cancer.*

I'm sorry to have to inform you of the above and that I have to hammer it home this way. But in my professional life, I am first and foremost a scientist. We work with research and facts, we present evidence, engage in study after study, and do all we can to dispute the findings of our contemporaries to come to safe and well-researched conclusions on what we are studying, be it new drugs or some alternative therapy that's all the rage. All conventional cancer treatments, such as chemotherapy and radiotherapy, must go through rigorous testing **by law** to prove that they work. And only after rigorous testing, which I discuss in the chapter on clinical trials, are new treatments approved by the Food and Drug Administration (FDA) and introduced into the populace. And then, they are introduced slowly and with a watchful eye on results and interactions. Most alternative therapies have not been through such testing, and again, there is no scientific evidence that they work.

Alternative therapies, like complementary treatment, can, and often do, interact with your conventional medical treatment. But in the case of alternative therapies, we find there are more chances for them to prove unsafe and cause harmful side effects. Not only are these therapies often tagged with that "natural" label and therefore thought to be harmless to the patient (and natural doesn't necessarily equal harmless), they are often more radical than complementary treatments and their claims wider reaching. It's a sad fact that, looking for a last vestige of hope, many cancer patients stop their traditional treatment altogether to sign on for exclusive, yet untested, alternate therapies. But be cautioned: ***giving up your conventional cancer treatment for an alternative therapy could reduce your chance of curing or controlling your cancer.***

Examples of alternative cancer therapies include:

- Laetrile
- Shark Cartilage
- Gerson Therapy

I know for my mother, all three times she came to battle cancer, CAMS was simply not on the table; these treatments and approaches weren't practiced or even discussed at her oncology clinic. My mother had the same doctor from her first cancer treatments, through her second diagnosis, and he wasn't necessarily the kind of doctor who was open to, or even knowledgeable about, anything other than the traditional treatments or trials out there. I wasn't even aware of anything beyond what I knew from my work, to tell you the truth.

Can I say with absolute certainty that I wouldn't have been tempted to give shark cartilage a try had it been presented to my mother as some sort of hope? I tend to think my background would have instilled a caution in me. But to be honest, during that last year of my mom's life, as the cancer spread to her brain and she underwent sheer hell (I still don't know how she managed through that!), I might have prompted her to try something that I normally would have mocked. You do get quite desperate to relieve the suffering of somebody you love or your own terrible sickness when you come to the last trying days of it.

I'll let Joyce weigh in here with her experience with this controversial subject:

> We hear of people either getting the wrong information and completely fraudulent care CAMs. As Deb says here, there are

plenty of things that work but lots that don't, but cancer patients will try to find hope. I knew of a young man who was diagnosed with a very rare form of cancer. He lived in quite a rural area of the country, so his options for treatment were few and what was being done for him wasn't responsive, and his cancer was progressing. He was twenty-six, had just had a baby; he was just starting his life, so you can believe he wanted to live a long, healthy life. At a point late in his treatment, he and his family found a doctor that offered hope—with an unapproved treatment. The physician claimed he had cured many people's cancer through a new radical treatment; it was unapproved, and the group of patients was limited to his practice—there were no large-scale clinical trials. This young man, pretty much seeing his mortality racing up at him all too quickly, was swayed to undergo this treatment; the poor guy was desperate. He wasn't cured.

This is an example of the bad side of CAMs.

But I do know for a fact, and there is plenty of proof that meditation, gentle yoga, and imagery have been known to positively affect the health and the possibilities for patients. Fear and anxiety levels can be managed, energy levels increased, and there is good brain-body research to support some of these practices. There is some great stuff out there, and CAM is also being actively investigated and recommended at large national cancer centers. The important point is, one has to find legitimate sources of information and research the facts through reliable, best-practices cancer providers.

It is very important to talk to your cancer doctor if you're considering any complementary or alternative therapies. He or she will be able to advise you on the safety of different types of approaches and what he or she feels could be effective . . . as well as what they feel could be dangerous. It's also important to let your complementary or alternative therapist know about your conventional cancer treatment. You have cancer; you need full disclosure at all times with any healthcare professional who is treating you, from your oncologist to the guy who's teaching you downward-facing dog.

Remember, real hope comes from getting reputable information and making your treatment decisions based on scientific facts. As we will see in the next chapter, it takes quite a bit of research, both in the lab and then with patient participation, to introduce a treatment into mainstream use. Even when a new drug or some new procedure is introduced, years before it becomes commonplace, researchers have gone through exacting measures to test it.

Therefore, the clinical trial, which we will get into in the next chapter.

Takeaways

- Explore the treatments available for your type of cancer.
- Prepare yourself, best you can, for the side effects that you will most likely have when undergoing certain treatments.
- Be very careful in engaging in CAMs (complementary and alternative therapies). Many have not been proven to help in cancer care and, in some cases, have been proven to be detrimental to cancer care.

RESOURCES:

The **National Cancer Institute**'s specific page on cancer treatment, https://www.cancer.gov/about-cancer/treatment 1-800-4-cancer.

American Cancer Society's specific page on cancer treatment, https://www.cancer.org/treatment/treatments-and-side-effects/treatment-types.html, 800-227-2345.

Natural Medicines Comprehensive Database, www.naturalmedicines-database.com, provides the largest number of evidence-based reviews on uses, safety, interactions, and dosage of a wide variety of natural medicines.

CAMS

American Cancer Society's alternate treatments page, https://www.cancer.org/treatment/treatments-and-side-effects/complementary-and-alternative-medicine.html.

National Center for Complementary and Alternative Medicine, www.nccam.nih.gov. The U.S. government's lead agency for scientific research on CAMs.

Cam-Cancer, http://www.cam-cancer.org/, an "open-access, nonprofit web resource" for health professionals looking to gain information and assist in CAM care.

Chapter 5

Is a Clinical Trial Right for Me?

I was out of the hospital two weeks after giving birth to my second son when my mother was diagnosed with breast cancer again. She and my father had been on vacation, and on the drive back my mother began feeling discomfort in her chest. At the time she put it down to the seatbelt annoying her during such a long car ride, but when she went in to get checked, her doctor found a lump in her remaining breast.

My mother had been cancer free for almost fifteen years, and we all thought she was cured. We found out later that this second tumor had probably been hiding out in her system for a while. Even though she had been on top of her regular checkups and yearly mammogram, there she was back for surgery, chemo, and then radiation therapy. Mom underwent all of it again and was again clear . . . this time for two years. Two years later was when they found that her cancer had metastasized, spreading through her body, growing in her rib, her collarbone, and her liver. Her second round of chemo two years before hadn't eradicated the cancer.

Now we were on the slow slide down the hill. This was something I was only too aware of, a fact my mother realized but we didn't speak about at all. She simply went on living her life. And it was during this third go-round that she stepped into clinical trials.

In the years between my mother first presenting when I was back in college and that third time when cancer would eventually take her life, medicines and treatments had advanced significantly. The medical community's overall knowledge about cancer had grown, and amazing discoveries seemed to be coming at us daily. Newer and better treatments, drugs, and procedures had been developed, and as science advanced, many treatments became less scattershot and even family histories could now highlight specific risks. While my grandmother and her sisters never had breast cancer, every one of their daughters died from the disease. My mom was concerned that there might be some genetic mutations in her DNA that were partly to blame for her cancer. She entered a genetic screening trial at this point (I'll explain what a screening trial is in a bit) to determine whether she had anything genetic that could have been passed on to my sisters and me that would put us at a higher risk of developing breast cancer. The results of her genetic test, thankfully, did not reveal any known genetic risks for her cancer, which was certainly a relief to her and us all, but maybe gave us a false sense of security as well. At the time, two genes were the focus of testing for breast cancer, but over the last ten years, we've learned of many other genes that can play a role. When my sister was diagnosed with breast cancer around the same age that my mom had originally been diagnosed, we weren't sure anymore that genetics wasn't involved. After talking with a genetic counselor, my sister and I both underwent genetic testing.

Although we never identified a genetic cause for my mother's cancer, by participating in this clinical trial, my mother felt like she was doing something to find answers and help protect my sisters and me. Certainly, she wanted more time with our family and would do everything she could to stay alive. But I also know Mom wanted to help others who would face the same diagnosis in the future. In fact, as it stands presently, there is some evidence to suggest that there may even be a genetic connection between the breast cancer my mother had and the melanoma I had. The research is far away from any concrete conclusions, but without clinical trials, this kind of finding, and many more that could make significant changes in cancer care, would simply not be found.

So, Should You Consider a Clinical Trial?

Depending on what type of cancer you have and the treatment options available to you, you may want to consider participating in a clinical trial. **Clinical trials are designed and conducted to answer questions and to further our knowledge about diseases and treatments.** If the recommended treatment available for your cancer is effective, there may still be clinical trials that seek to improve upon it, or trials that evaluate ways to improve how you feel during treatment. These trials can be available close to where you live, or they may be halfway around the world from you. While clinical trials may be funded or sponsored by any number of sources, including hospitals, companies, or the government, they are developed by panels of experts and investigators, often from various fields, to ensure that they are in the best interest of patients and are able to answer the questions they are designed to answer.

Participating in this extra step is not for everyone, and a patient's reasons for participating in a clinical trial run from deeply personal ones like my mom's, to curiosity and not wanting to leave any stone unturned. Perhaps your doctor has recommended you consider a clinical trial (my mom's doctor initially came to my mom about participating), or you have found a clinical trial while researching across the Internet. While clinical trials may seem scary, in fact, many patients who participate in clinical trials feel that they are getting even more attention from their doctors and nurses, and better care than they might outside of a clinical trial.

Participating in a clinical trial offers many potential benefits:

- Having access to a potentially better treatment option for your particular type of cancer
- A chance to improve how you feel during and possibly after treatment
- Helping doctors develop new treatments that may benefit you and others who also have cancer

In my work, I find that the typical cancer patient these days is quite well educated, or firmly on their way to being so after they find out they have cancer. Scores of sites to research across the Internet will not only list what trials are currently being conducted but which ones are beginning in the near future. In addition, many patient advocacy groups on the web help match patients to a trial; patients are matched through criteria such as what kind of cancer they have and where in the country they happen to live. Many patients simply won't accept a "no option left" diagnosis and take it upon themselves to search out these trials where they might indeed find their last best hope or at least feel empowered to try.

Clinical trials are developed to answer specific questions about a new drug, treatment, or test; first and foremost, they look to determine the new drug or treatment's efficacy and safety, or in the case of a test, how consistent the results are and how predictive the method is. In the end, scientists want to know if what they are developing will help a patient suffering from a particular disease; if the drug or treatment is effective in making tumors smaller, prolonging the life of patients; or even if it will minimize the side effects patients experience. Because each trial is developed to answer specific questions (also referred to as "endpoints"), the number of individuals (often referred to as "subjects") involved, and the types of tests and treatments involved will be unique to each clinical trial. Here are a few examples of the different types of clinical trials that you may see:

<u>Treatment Trials:</u> These trials test new kinds of treatments for your particular type of cancer. They can include surgery, radiation, chemotherapy, immunotherapy, or biologic/vaccine therapy. The questions asked by these trials include whether the therapy is able to reduce the size of the cancer (called "response rate"), whether it can lengthen the amount of time during and after the treatment that a patient lives with the cancer but it does not get worse ("progression free survival"), or if a patient will live longer after the start of treatment (overall survival).

<u>Supportive Care Trials:</u> These trials evaluate new ways to make you more comfortable and improve your quality of life when you have cancer. Examples of these trials would be new pain medicines, new anti-nausea drugs, or therapies that strengthen your immune system by increasing certain types of blood cell production. Endpoints for these trials may include the ability to reduce the severity or frequency of a particular effect (such as pain, or nausea and vomiting), or reducing complications associated with treatment (such as infection or anemia). Often these trials will include information reported directly by the patient ("Patient Reported Outcomes") that may be collected through diaries or questions asked at your clinic visits or even through technology such as smart phones.

<u>Diagnostic Marker Trials:</u> These trials focus on finding new ways to detect and understand diseases such as cancer. They could include new approaches to body scans or blood tests that can detect certain things within your body. There are three general types of markers:

Diagnostic markers can help assess where cancer started (tissue of origin) or the specific subtype of a tumor. *Prognostic markers* are used to determine the likelihood of what will happen with your cancer and treatment (i.e. is your tumor likely to come back) regardless of the specific treatment you receive. One example is whether cancer cells have spread to lymph nodes in patients with solid tumors. If cancer has spread to lymph nodes, the chance the tumor will recur increases. *Predictive markers* help indicate the likelihood that a tumor will respond to a specific therapy. For example, breast cancers that express the estrogen receptor tend to respond to hormonal therapies such as tamoxifen.

Prevention Trials: These trials are done with a large group of people who are healthy and don't have cancer already, and are focused on finding better ways to prevent or lower the chances that people will get cancer. In some studies, people are asked to *do* something to lower cancer risk, like follow a special diet. In other cases, people are asked to *take* something to lower cancer risk, like vitamins. These could also include vaccines, exercise, or other lifestyle changes.

Screening Trials: These trials look for ways to detect certain types of cancer. For example, certain genetic changes can greatly increase the chances of developing breast cancer. This was the first type of clinical trial my mom participated in—genetic testing done to determine if there were any changes in her DNA that were causing her cancer or would put other families with similar DNA at higher risk.

Even for those people who want to participate in a clinical trial, and even meet the criteria for a particular trial, participation is not always easy. Sometimes doctors simply do not have the time to engage in a trial themselves or may not have the knowledge of possible clinical trials available to even suggest a patient go somewhere else to take part. For many patients, the process of reading all the information about a clinical trial (see at the end of this chapter) and deciding whether or not you want to participate (a daunting task in and of itself when you are not feeling your best) is overwhelming enough to make them feel like it's not worth it to participate.

As with all the decisions you make with your cancer treatment, participating in a clinical trial is something to weigh considerably and consult your doctor on, even if you do fit the criteria of the study.

The Steps to New Therapies

Developing a new therapy takes many years and requires several steps in the clinical trial process. Long before clinical trials can be started in humans, a tremendous amount of research has already been done in what are called "preclinical studies." Preclinical studies include in vitro (test tube or cell culture) and in vivo (animal) tests done to gather preliminary efficacy, toxicity, and safety information. Once these preclinical studies have been completed, an application is submitted to a regulatory agency such as the Food and Drug Administration (FDA) in the U.S. to determine if it is reasonably safe to start clinical trials in humans. When clinical trials are started in humans, researchers follow several steps (called "phases") to gather enough information first on the safety of a new therapy and then on whether the therapy can affect the cancer in individuals.

Phase I, the first step, is focused on understanding the proper dosage of a drug and how the therapy will be administered (by injection or orally). Patients in this phase are monitored closely for side effects, and additional tests may be required to assess how safe the proposed therapy is. These studies are very small, sometimes including only fifteen to thirty patients. Most Phase I studies are open to patients whose cancer has not responded to other therapies and for which other known options are not available. For this reason, patients in a Phase I trial are probably not undergoing any other treatment at the time.

Once researchers have determined how the new therapy should be administered and the best dose, a Phase II study will begin.

Phase II studies gather more information on safety, as well as what benefits the new treatment provides to patients. In this phase, researchers determine what effect the specific treatment being studied has on the cancer or the side effect being studied. These studies are again fairly small and may only include forty to one hundred patients. Phase II studies may be open to patients who may or may not have received previous therapy for their cancer, who still have other treatment options available, or who have halted their previous treatment.

Notice that as the clinical trial process continues, even though more specifics are known about a treatment, and therefore patients with a more specified type of cancer may be sought, the population size increases for test subjects.

Phase III: Once a new therapy has been demonstrated to have a benefit to patients, and for a specific kind of cancer, it will be tested against another treatment option currently being used. The goal of these studies is to simply determine if one treatment is better than another, or if one perhaps causes fewer side effects than another. Depending on the questions being answered by the study, hundreds or even thousands of patients may be required to participate, including patients newly diagnosed with cancer who often have other treatment options available to them when they decide to participate in a Phase III study.

This was when my mother came into her second clinical trial, a Phase III trial.

Two and a half years after her second diagnosis, mastectomy, and treatment for that lump found in her remaining breast, my mother began feeling a sharp pain in her ribs. A scan at that time found another tumor there, as well as one in her collarbone. It was the same breast cancer spreading, presenting as tumors and floating around in her bloodstream looking for somewhere to land next; the chemo from two years earlier had not eradicated it. Since removing the tumors once her cancer spread was not an option, my mother was yet again put on chemotherapy. But Mom's doctor wasn't so pleased with the side effects and results from this treatment, so she got into a Phase III clinical trial testing a monoclonal antibody. Over the span of years that my mom was diagnosed and treated, her cancer had changed in that she was now showing positive for a certain marker that made her a candidate for this biological treatment. In this Phase III clinical trial, a new therapy was being added onto existing treatments to determine if this new therapy added benefit to the usual standard care.

Did her participation in the trial prolong or better the quality of my mother's life those last few years she had left? I think it prolonged her life for a bit . . . maybe a couple of months, and certainly it kept our hope alive. I wanted my mom around for as long as I could have her alive, and as I say, even though the end was difficult, she kept on living life. If my mom hadn't been an inspiration before, she certainly was during those last few months of her battle.

At the end of each clinical trial, the researches share their results with the medical community at large. These days the results may be published online, presented at scientific meetings, or published in medical and scientific journals. This public airing allows further examination of the trial's findings and invites scrutiny—and even more study—by the scientific community at large. This major tenet of all scientific development is an important difference between alternative treatments and true studied cancer care. It is part and parcel of scientific study for other scientists to try and poke holes in the research of their contemporaries, run double blind tests, and attack findings from every angle. Such scrutiny proves that when new therapies or drugs are developed, they have been given a once, twice, thrice over, under the most exacting examination.

Even studies that don't lead to new treatments can still offer valuable insights.

In the U.S., the Food and Drug Administration (FDA) passed section 801 of Food and Drug Administration Amendments Act, FDAAA 801, which requires clinical trials started after September 2007 to be registered on a clinical trial registry data bank (such as clinicaltrials.gov) and to have those results posted once they are available. In the United States, the FDA is responsible for evaluating the results of clinical trials to determine if a new therapy should be approved for use. But even after a new therapy is approved and after the rigorous approval of the FDA, additional clinical trials may be conducted in order to monitor long-term safety and effectiveness. These Phase IV studies are sometimes referred to as **post-marketing studies,** as the FDA has already approved the therapy for use.

Phase IV might include the same number of patients as a Phase III or even more, but these last tests tend to be broader in scope, pushing to evaluate the new drug in a real world setting, beyond the controlled clinical trial. Physicians working with cancer patients daily, both in small offices and big hospital facilities, administer the newly approved drug on patients who are then monitored closely. What they eventually hope for, of course, is to find something that becomes a better standard of care from what was used before.

Time and again, drugs found through clinical trials have become standard bearers for cancer treatment, completely revolutionizing treatment.

What to Expect if You Are Considering a Clinical Trial

Before a doctor can open a clinical trial at his/her office/hospital, an Institutional Review Board (IRB) will first evaluate the study to ensure that is designed well, that the questions that need to be answered can indeed be answered, and that patients will be appropriately informed on what to expect. The IRB is a committee established to protect the rights and welfare of human research subjects. The committee is comprised of at least five members, including at least one scientist and one non-scientist, and possibly a patient advocate, who conduct formal review of clinical trials and make the determination on whether the trial is approved to be conducted at a particular clinic/hospital.

If you want to consider participating in a clinical trial, it is important to understand the steps involved here. Each clinical trial has a set of criteria that describe the type of patients eligible for the study ("eligibility criteria" or "inclusion criteria"); the focus of these criteria is to ensure patient safety. These criteria may include factors such as your age, the type of cancer you have, other medical conditions you have, medicines you are taking, or treatment you have already received for your cancer. Your doctor or research nurse will ask you questions about your health that will be used to determine if you are eligible to participate. If you *are* eligible, you will then be provided with additional information on the trial and what to expect if you participate. All patients who are involved in a clinical study must sign an *informed* written consent. This contract proves that the patient understands what their treatment will entail and what rights they have throughout the study. The "informed" part here is most important for patients potentially embarking on a clinical trial, as they need to be informed of:

• the fact that the clinical trial they are participating in might not benefit their health at all

- the multitude of unknown risks they could be exposing themselves to by participating in the trial, as well as the potential of unknown side effects or discomforts they may experience
- the protocols of the trial and what will be done, as well as what is expected from them in their participation
- in participating in the clinical trial, they may be engaging in procedures that could be quite different than in typical cancer treatments
- the agreement they are entering into that their participation in this clinical trial is voluntary

A patient always has the right to remove their consent at any time, regardless of reason. And it behooves those hoping to embark on a trial of this nature to ask their healthcare team questions at all times during the process. According to the Food and Drug Administration, the informed consent process must provide "sufficient opportunity for the participant to consider whether to participate." The FDA considers this to include allowing sufficient time for participants to consider the information and time, and opportunity, for the participant to ask questions and have those questions answered.

The investigator (or other study staff who are conducting the informed consent interview) and the participant should exchange information and discuss the contents of the informed consent document. This process must occur under circumstances that minimize the possibility of coercion or undue influence. Consent forms can be quite long and provide quite a bit of information for you to review. In some cases, patients will need to review and sign more than one consent form for a clinical trial. So that you have an idea of what to expect, an example of what is included in an informed consent form is provided below. It is based on the template that has been developed by the National Cancer Institute (NCI).

x x x x x x x x x x x x x x x x x x x x x x x x

What is the usual approach to my type of cancer?

This section will outline what type of cancer you have and how people are usually treated. For a treatment trial, this would include information on surgery, chemotherapy, and/or radiation therapy that you would normally receive. This section will also outline what treatments have been approved for your type of cancer. Last, there will be information on how patients who get the standard treatment usually do (i.e. how many patients are cancer free at five years).

What are my other choices if I do not take part in this study?

If you decide not to take part in this study, you have other choices. These will be outlined clearly. For example:

- You may choose to have the usual approach described above.
- You may choose to take part in a different study, if one is available.
- Or you may choose not to be treated for cancer (as appropriate, consider adding) but you may want to receive comfort care to relieve symptoms.

Why is this study being done?

The purpose of the study, or the questions being asked by the study, will be outlined. Examples may include:

- Compare any good and bad effects of using a new therapy *along with* the standard treatment to the standard treatment alone.

- Test the ability of the new therapy to extend your life beyond what is expected with standard treatment,
- Test the ability of the new treatment to reduce the bad effects of standard treatment.

This section should also provide information on the expected size or number of people taking part in the study.

What are the study groups?

This section will outline the design of the study.

- Is it a randomized study where a computer will by chance assign you to one of the groups in the study? If so, what are the different treatment groups, and what are the chances of your being assigned to any particular one?
- Is it a single-arm study, where all patients receive access to the same therapy?

How long will I be in this study?

This section will describe the intervention or treatment you will be receiving, how long you will receive treatment, and how long your doctor will continue to watch you for side effects and follow your condition.

What extra tests and procedures will I have if I take part in this study?

This section will include a list of exams, tests, and procedures that are NOT a part of the standard approach, or those that will be done more frequently than usual.

- Before starting the study, you may need extra tests or *procedures* to find out if you can participate in the study. These could include blood tests, additional scans, or other tests.

- During the study you may need extra mandatory tests or procedures so the answers to the questions being asked by the study can be answered.

  ◊ Specimens may be collected (tissue collected during biopsy, blood samples, urine samples), including a description about how the specimen will be used, as well as any potential risks associated with the specimen collection.

  ◊ If any specimens that are collected will be stored for biobanking, this will be explained and discussed further, usually in the section on "optional studies."

  ◊ Additional scans (CT scans, bone scans, etc.) may also be required.

  ◊ A calendar or statement outlining how often these tests and procedures will be done will also be included.

- A description of how your privacy will be protected with regards to test results should be included, as well as whether the results will be available to you or your doctor.

In most cases, if not all, neither you nor your healthcare plan/insurance carrier should be billed for these extra tests and procedures required by the study.

What possible risks can I expect from taking part in this study?

This section should outline foreseeable risks and discomforts that are not physical side effects. Examples may include:

- You may lose time at work or home and spend more time in the hospital or doctor's office than usual.

- You may be asked sensitive or private questions which you normally do not discuss.

- If the study is randomized: The study drug(s)/study approach may not be better, and could possibly be worse, than the usual approach for your cancer.

- If the study includes genetic testing: There is a risk someone could get access to the personal information in your medical records or other information researchers have kept about you. Someone might be able to trace this information back to you. The researchers believe the chance that someone will identify you is quite small, but the risk may change in the future as people come up with new ways of tracing information. In some cases, this information could be used to make it harder for you to get or keep a job. (For non–U.S. participants, please verify the existence of such laws before including the following sentence.) There are laws against misuse of genetic information, but they may not give full protection. The researchers believe the chance these things will happen is very small, but cannot promise that they will not occur.

- The specific therapy used in this study may affect how different parts of your body work such as your liver, kidneys, heart, and blood. The study doctor will be testing your blood and will let you know if changes occur that may affect your health.

- There is also a risk that you could have side effects from the study drug(s)/study approach. Here are important points about side effects:

- The study doctors do not know who will or will not have side effects.

- Some side effects may go away soon, some may last a long time, or some may never go away.
- Some side effects may interfere with your ability to have children.
- Some side effects may be serious and may even result in death.

Here are important points about how you and the study doctor can make side effects less of a problem:

- Tell the study doctor if you notice or feel anything different so they can see if you are having a side effect.
- The study doctor may be able to treat some side effects.
- The study doctor may adjust the study drugs to try to reduce side effects.

There will also be information included that shows the most common and the most serious side effects that researchers know about. There might be other side effects that researchers do not yet know about. If important new side effects are found, the study doctor will discuss these with you.

What possible benefits can I expect from taking part in this study?

It is not always known what the possible benefits of the study are, but there will be information included in this section to clarify what they may be, or even if it is not possible to know at this time if there are any benefits.

Can I stop taking part in this study?

Yes. You can decide to stop at any time. If you decide to stop for any reason, it is important to let the study doctor know as soon as possible so you can stop safely. If you stop, you can decide whether to let the study doctor continue to provide your medical information to the organization running the study.

The study doctor will tell you about new information or changes in the study that may affect your health or willingness to continue in the study.

The study doctor may take you out of the study:

- If your health changes and the study is no longer in your best interest
- If new information becomes available
- If you do not follow the study rules
- If the study is stopped by the sponsor, IRB, or the FDA.

What are my rights in this study?

Taking part in this study is your choice. No matter what decision you make, and even if your decision changes, there will be no penalty to you. You will not lose medical care or any legal rights.

For questions about your rights while in this study, call the _____ *(insert name of center)* Institutional Review Board at _____ *(insert telephone number).*

What are the costs of taking part in this study?

This section will provide information and clarification on what will be provided at no charge to you, and what costs will need to be paid by you and/or your health insurance company. Before you decide to be in the study, you should check with your health plan or insurance company to find out exactly what they will pay for.

If there is any compensation for your participation or reimbursement for expenses, this will be clearly outlined in this section.

What happens if I am injured or hurt because I took part in this study?

This section outlines whether the study sponsor will offer to pay for medical treatment for any injury that results from taking part in the study. If you are injured or hurt as a result of taking part in a study and need medical treatment, make sure to tell your study doctor. Your insurance company may not be willing to pay for study-related injury. If you have no insurance, you would be responsible for any costs.

Who will see my medical information?

This section will outline your privacy as it relates to your medical information. Your information may be given out if required by law. For example, certain states require doctors to report to health boards if they find a disease like tuberculosis. However, researchers do their best to make sure that any information released will not identify you. Some of your health information, and/or information about your specimen, from a study may be kept in a central database for research. Your name or contact information will not be put in the database.

There are organizations that may inspect your records. These organizations are required to make sure your information is kept private, unless required by law to provide information. Some of these organizations are:

• The study sponsor and any drug company supporting the study

- The Institutional Review Board, IRB, is a group of people who review the research with the goal of protecting the people who take part in the study.
- The Food and Drug Administration and the National Cancer Institute in the U.S., and similar ones if other countries are involved in the study.

Where can I get more information?

U.S. law requires that information on clinical trials is available online. You should be able to find a description of your specific clinical trial on http://www.ClinicalTrials.gov. This website will not include information that can identify you. At most, the website will include a summary of the results. You can search this website at any time.

Who can answer my questions about this study?

You can talk to the study doctor about any questions or concerns you have about this study or to report side effects or injuries. Contact the study doctor _____ *(insert name of study doctor[s])* at _____ *(insert telephone number).*

ADDITIONAL STUDIES SECTION

This section will include information about optional studies you can choose to take part in.

This part of the consent form is about optional studies that you can choose to take part in. While you will not get health benefits from any of these studies, the researchers hope the results of the optional studies will help other people with cancer in the future.

It will be clarified if the results will/will not be added to your medical records and if you or your study doctor will/will not know the results.

You will not be billed for these optional studies. You can still take part in the main study even if you say no to any or all of these studies. If you sign up for but cannot complete any of the studies for any reason, you can still take part in the main study.

Circle your choice of "yes" or "no" for each of the following studies.

1. Optional imaging study

This could include an extra scan (one that is already used in medical care but it would be taken at a time point in your treatment that is not usual) or an investigational scan (one that is being studied to determine how accurate and useful it may be). Information on what the scan would be used for, what would be involved, and the potential risks would also be provided.

Please circle your answer: I choose to take part in the imaging study:

YES   NO

2. Optional Quality of Life Study

If you choose to take part in this study, you will be asked to fill out a form with questions about your emotional or physical well-being. Researchers will use this information to *learn more about how cancer and cancer treatment affects people.*

Information outlining how often you would need to complete the form, how long it will take to complete the form, and the types of questions that will be asked will be provided.

Please circle your answer: I choose to take part in the Quality of Life study and will fill out these forms:

YES   NO

3. Optional Sample Collections for Laboratory Studies and/or Bio-banking for Possible Future Studies

Researchers are trying to learn more about cancer. Much of this research is done using samples from cancer patients' tissue, blood, urine, or other fluids. Through these studies, researchers hope to find new ways to prevent, detect, treat, or cure cancer.

Some of these studies may be about genes. Genes carry information about features that are found in you and in people who are related to you. Researchers are interested in the way genes affect how your body responds to treatment.

Information about the specific sample requirements and how the samples will be used and/or stored will be provided in this section. The researchers will ask your permission to store and use your samples and related health information (for example, your response to cancer treatment, results of study tests and medicines you are given) for medical research. Storing samples for future studies is called "biobanking." Information on where these samples will be stored will also be provided.

WHAT IS INVOLVED?

If you agree to take part, here is what will happen next:

1. *A sample will be collected (this section will outline what the sample is and how it will be collected).*

- Your sample and some related health information will be sent to a researcher for use in the study described above. Remaining samples may be stored in the biobank, along with samples from other people who take part. The samples will be kept until they are used up.

2. Qualified researchers can submit a request to use the materials stored in the biobanks. A science committee at the clinical trials organization will review each request. There will also be an ethics review to ensure that the request is necessary and proper. Researchers will not be given your name or any other information that could directly identify you.

3. Neither you nor your study doctor will be notified when research will be conducted or given reports or other information about any research that is done using your samples.

4. Some of your genetic and health information may be placed in central databases that may be public, along with information from many other people. Information that could directly identify you will not be included.

WHAT ARE THE POSSIBLE RISKS?

1. There is a risk that someone could get access to the personal information in your medical records or other information researchers have stored about you.

2. There is a risk that someone could trace the information in a central database back to you. Even without your name or other identifiers, your genetic information is unique to you. The researchers believe the chance that someone will identify you is very small, but the

risk may change in the future as people come up with new ways of tracing information.

3. In some cases, this information could be used to make it harder for you to get or keep a job or insurance. There are laws against the misuse of genetic information, but they may not give full protection. There can also be a risk in knowing genetic information. New health information about inherited traits that might affect you or your blood relatives could be found during a study. The researchers believe the chance these things will happen is very small, but cannot promise that they will not occur.

HOW WILL INFORMATION ABOUT ME BE KEPT PRIVATE?

Your privacy is very important to the researchers, and they will make every effort to protect it. Here are a few of the steps they will take:

1. When your sample(s) is sent to the researchers, no information identifying you (such as your name) will be sent. Samples will be identified by a unique code only.

2. The list that links the unique code to your name will be kept separate from your sample and health information. Any biobank and/or clinical research staff with access to the list must sign an agreement to keep your identity confidential.

3. Information that identifies you will not be given to anyone, unless required by law.

4. If research results are published, your name and other personal information will not be used.

WHAT ARE THE POSSIBLE BENEFITS?

Your samples may be helpful to research. The researchers, using the samples from you and others, might make discoveries that could help people in the future.

ARE THERE ANY COSTS OR PAYMENTS?

There are no costs to you or your insurance. You will not be paid for taking part. If any of the research leads to new tests, drugs, or other commercial products, you will not share in any profits.

WHAT IF I CHANGE MY MIND?

If you decide you no longer want your samples to be used, you can call the study doctor, _____, *(insert name of study doctor for main trial)* at _____ *(insert telephone number of study doctor for main trial),* who will let the researchers know. Then, any sample that remains in the bank will no longer be used, and related health information will no longer be collected. Samples or related information that have already been given to or used by researchers will not be returned.

WHAT IF I HAVE MORE QUESTIONS?

If you have questions about the use of your samples for research, contact the study doctor, _____, *(insert name of study doctor for main trial)*, at _____ *(insert telephone number of study doctor for main trial).*

Please circle your answer to show whether or not you would like to take part in each:

SAMPLES FOR THE LABORATORY STUDIES:

I agree to have my specimen collected, and I agree that my specimen sample(s) and related information may be used for the laboratory study(ies) described above.

YES   NO

I agree that my study doctor, or their representative, may contact me or my physician to see if I wish to learn about results from this(ese) study(ies).

YES   NO

SAMPLES FOR FUTURE RESEARCH STUDIES:

My samples and related information may be kept in a biobank for use in future health research.

YES   NO

I agree that my study doctor, or their representative, may contact me or my physician to see if I wish to participate in other research in the future.

YES   NO

This is the end of the section about optional studies.

My Signature Agreeing to Take Part in the Main Study

I have read this consent form or had it read to me. I have discussed it with the study doctor and my questions have been answered. I will be given a signed copy of this form. I agree to take part in the main study *and any additional studies where I circled yes.*

Participant's signature_____

Date of signature_____

Signature of person(s) conducting the informed consent discussion _____

_____

Date of signature_____

x x x x x x x x x x x x x x x x x x x x x x x x

If the patient is a minor and too young to give informed consent but old enough to understand the proposed clinical trial and expected risks and benefits, then they will be asked to provide their "assent" to the clinical trial, expressing their willingness to participate. While assent to participate in a clinical trial is not always required by law, many IRBs may require it, with age requirements depending on the institution and the specific clinical trial. The following outlines the assent process:

- Parents or guardians first give their informed permission for their child to participate in the clinical trial. Usually both parents will need to give their permission, except in cases where one parent has died, is unknown, is incompetent, or has sole legal custody.

- Once informed consent has been given, the research team will explain the trial to the child in language that he/she can understand. This will include information on what it means to take part in the trial, and what the child can expect.

- Often the research team will use visual aids in addition to written information to help explain the information.

- Throughout the process, the child should be encouraged to ask questions.

Participating in a clinical trial (if you are eligible) is a personal decision. I have revealed my mother's motivations. You might share in some of her reasons, have a few of your own, or over time conclude that although you first wanted to participate in a trial, on deeper reflection, you don't want to. In some cases, and this was certainly true for my mother, patients may have no other option for hope of beating their cancer, so they do indeed jump into the trial with as much enthusiasm as they can muster, sick as they might be.

Depending on a whole host of mundane factors like those mentioned in chapter 3 on how/where to find a doctor, sometimes even the distance a patient has to travel for a trial makes it too difficult for them to participate. I think it behooves you to at least explore all options of treatments available to you, consider those that are scientifically sound and being researched in the manner I have outlined above, and proceed—or not—according to what your heart tells you.

Takeaways

- Clinical trials are available and happening all the time for a whole host of treatments and drugs.
- While a patient's reason(s) for participating in a clinical trial will vary, it is important to understand what questions each trial is looking to answer and what will be required.
- Remember, if you find a clinical trial that seems to be a good fit for you, you must match specific criteria before you can be included in a specific trial.
- Each patient must also fill out an informed consent form before they can be considered for a clinical trial. This is strictly for the patient's safety and complete understanding of what they are volunteering for.

- Patients who are minors but who are old enough to understand information about the clinical trial will need to provide their assent before they will be able to participate.

RESOURCES:

The **ACS Clinical Trial Matching Service**, https://www.cancer.org/
treatment/treatments-and-side-effects/clinical-trials/clinical-trials-matching-
service-find-trial.html, 800-303-5691, offers a free, confidential program
for patients, their families, and healthcare workers to find cancer clinical
trials most appropriate to a patient's medical and personal situation.

The **National Cancer Institute**'s page on clinical trials: https://www.cancer.
gov/about-cancer/treatment/clinical-trials/patient-safety/childrens-assent.
This includes a section for pediatric clinical trials as well.

The **Food and Drug Administration**'s **(FDA)** site for informed consent
for clinical trials: https://www.fda.gov/ForPatients/ClinicalTrials/Informed-
Consent/default.htm.

The **U.S. National Library of Medicine (U.S.N.L.M)**, http://www.Clini-
calTrials.gov, is a massive database for patients and their families to search
through current clinical trials via specific criteria.

Chapter 6

The Business of Your Health —Health Insurance, Legal

Up until this point, I have been sticking to the medical aspect of cancer care. I've had Philip, LeAnn, and Joyce give their answers to the big question of the first thing you should do after you're diagnosed, and you've seen them weigh in other places in the book (as they will again). I have sprinkled in my life experiences when I thought they'd make things clearer, but really, I want now to address the actual "in the trenches" details of being diagnosed and considering your treatment options. I hope the first few chapters above help in this most difficult time in your life. But while your type of cancer, its treatment, possible clinical trials, and what questions to ask about it all are foremost concerns, I'd be remiss in what I am trying to offer here if I don't discuss the *business* of your health.

As Phil says:

Would it not be a better world if those of us affected by this life-threatening disease did not have to worry that our lives would be further threatened by financial ruin and stress? Unfortunately, health insurance coverage of cancer care is top of mind for almost all patients. Why? Well, for one thing, the popular press has covered this problem and provided personal stories of how cancer care has bankrupted individuals. For another, I have read academic studies that describe the financial stress that a diagnosis of cancer unleashes, suggesting that bankruptcy may predispose death. It is extremely important to talk about insurance and finances when talking about cancer.

⊚≋⊚

When my mother was first diagnosed with cancer back in 1989, she and my father were both working and had good insurance coverage. She did her best not to miss too much work, scheduling chemotherapy treatments later in the week so she would feel worse over the weekend and could go back to work on that following Monday. We were lucky in that her diagnosis and treatment did not cause any real financial strains on our family. However, once she was diagnosed, she would be unable to get healthcare insurance outside of what was provided by an employer, because she now had a "preexisting condition" and was deemed to be too high of a risk. Later, when my parents reached retirement age, part of the decision as to when my father could retire was based on having the insurance to cover my mother until she reached Medicare age and could get some coverage that way. Medicare won't restrict insurance coverage if a patient has a preexisting condition.

I was also lucky that I had a good job and health insurance when I was diagnosed with cancer. However, years later, when I decided to leave the rat race of corporate America to start my own consulting company, I soon learned that I had no way to get health insurance. Even though my cancer had been diagnosed nine years previously and I'd had no health issues since (for all intents and purposes I was cancer free), every insurance company I applied to denied me. I eventually went back into corporate America, partly to get access to health insurance.

Things are different now since the passing of the Patient Protection and Affordable Care Act (better known as the Affordable Care Act or

"Obamacare") in 2010. Insurance companies are now prevented (in some way) from denying anyone health insurance because of preexisting conditions. People have varying perspectives on the Affordable Care Act, and as of this writing there are many questions about what healthcare will look like in the future. It's not surprising that plenty of people don't understand health insurance or struggle to evaluate what they need, where to find it, and how to pay for it.

Really, what's happened to the healthcare industry in this country over the past decade would leave even the savviest health insurance CEO dizzy. I am constantly trying to make heads or tails of what is available for my family and me and trying to anticipate what might be coming down the pike. It all leaves me scratching my head when I try and research the ever-changing landscape, and I am in the healthcare business!

Even for the person with no true medical issues, health insurance can be a mountain to climb.

Let me try to untangle what you might be facing as a cancer patient—what insurance means to you, what precautions you need to be taking, and, in the end, what you can and cannot expect from your state and our government when it comes to your rights and protections. I will also attempt to give you a leg up on some of what you might face with legal questions that could arise over your care.

The financial burdens of cancer—treatment bills, loss of work time, figuring exactly what your insurance will or will not pay for—can present unique challenges. And then there are the many men and women who do not have insurance; what do they do?

Know What You Know and Find Out What You Don't

Even with the changes brought about by the Affordable Care Act, many individuals and families may not have health insurance. So, what happens if you don't have health insurance and you are diagnosed with cancer? Will you be able to get any treatment? The good news is that there are government and private organizations that may be able to help. The bad news is that it will likely take time and effort to work through the system, and you may need help from your support system to navigate through everything. Here are my recommendations for organizations that you should contact for assistance:

- The National Cancer Institute's (NCI) Cancer Information Service has information on how to get free screening tests (mammograms, pap smears, etc.) and treatment (1-800-4-CANCER or 1-800-422-6237).
- Your local Department of Health and Human Services will be able to help determine if you are eligible for Medicaid or other programs.
- Call your local hospital and ask to speak with a social worker. Find out any information you can about "charity care" or "indigent programs."
- Certain hospitals in the U.S. are required to provide treatment to patients who can't afford to pay for their care. Approximately three hundred hospitals receive funds from the government, and under the Hill-Burton Act, these hospitals must treat patients regardless of their ability to pay.
- Pharmaceutical companies often establish programs that help patients with the cost of treatments. These may include help with insurance reimbursement, discounted or free medications for patients who do not qualify for other assistance, or referrals to co-pay relief programs. Contact the Partnership for Prescription Assistance (PPA), or have your doctor's office contact them for you: www.pparx.org, (888-477-2669).

- The National Breast and Cervical Cancer Early Detection Program (NBCCEDP) runs a prescreening program with the Centers for Disease Control and Prevention (CDC). It helps give low-income, the uninsured, and so many other women the opportunity for breast and cervical cancer screening.
- You may need help with other expenses, like transportation, homecare, or childcare. Several organizations can help with these expenses. The Patient Advocate Foundation and the American Cancer Society are two organizations to contact.

If You Have Health Insurance

The best course of action with your health insurance, as is true of your overall health, is to be proactive. If cancer becomes part of your life, the best way to know how, where, if, and when your insurance is applicable is to explore the kind of coverage you have and what you can, and cannot, expect of it. A whole host of potential issues (issues you do not want nor will you be able to deal with as you become sicker or undergo treatment) can be avoided if you know exactly how you are covered and how best to initiate your policy's procedures. By nature, I am less a cynic than I am a realist. I wouldn't ever accuse insurance companies of being slow to pay or hoping you make a mistake on your end so they could bury you in paperwork. However, a form not filled out completely, some numbers transposed here and there, or a procedure not preapproved often won't see a patient or provider getting paid for a long time. Tracking down duplicate payments, checks sent to the wrong provider, determining what should have been paid for and wasn't . . . well, if you can avoid bureaucratic finagling and collection agencies calling, you will certainly feel less stress.

It should be apparent, then, that you should not only know what kind of policy you have—but know it well.

Luckily, with competition so fierce these days across the various private insurance companies, and ever since the implementation of and seemingly constant debate over the Affordable Healthcare Act, my experience has been that the general public is trying to get more informed over what they have and what they don't when it comes to their health insurance. As a nation, we seem to be engaging in a constant conversation about insurance and seem to be ever more aware of it. Again, things are bound to change soon or have already as of the writing of this book, but at least we all seem to be looking around a lot more and asking the questions about our present healthcare system.

In broad strokes, there are three types of healthcare plan options for the individual: HMOs, PPOs, and POSs. HMOs fall into two categories: Independent Physician Associations (IPAs) and stand-alone facilities. IPA physicians see patients in their offices as well as occasionally joining with other healthcare providers to form groups. The best known of these are Blue Cross, Blue Shield, and Aetna, names I am sure you have heard. Stand-alone facilities are the hospitals that provide all care within that HMO's facilities; Kaiser Permanente is one of the better-known stand-alones in this field.

PPOs, or Preferred Provider Organizations, are a group of healthcare providers who have joined together to provide their services to a specific insurance company at a reduced rate. POS, or Point of Service Plan, combines the HMO and the PPO. Members here decide when they want to use either the HMO or PPO part of their plan, often with different financial implications.

As you would expect, each of the above has specific advantages and disadvantages. If you have one of these plans already, I am sure you are aware of what you can and cannot do within your plan (or as I am suggesting here, you should get familiar with what you can and cannot do). For those looking to possibly switch their insurance or those without any insurance looking to get into either a POS, HMO, or PPO, do your research with all three types to see which might fit you best. There are many factors to consider, for both you and your family; concerns can range from your age, preexisting conditions, family genetics, even where in the country you live.

For those people who have healthcare through their employer, you still should get well acquainted with your healthcare plan's parameters. Don't rely on an HR person at the office to be coming down soon to educate you. Healthcare for something like cancer is not something we generally ever consider when we first sign up for a policy (at work or not), and, given the disease, it can come to tax a policy to its maximum. Play it safe and become familiar with your work policy, even if you are 100% healthy.

You need to understand whether your work health plan is insured or self-funded. Often a third party is involved in a self-funded plan, as employers enlist a third party, quite often an insurance company, to manage the plan. These third parties, often referred to as ASOs or Administrative Service Organizations, engage in the business side of things—claim processing, networking, etc.—but the employer is responsible for all liabilities and claims. This is certainly something that's good to know if and when you are trying to locate money your provider is asking you for or you have a bill needing to be paid.

Right now *is* the time to see that HR Department rep. They should be able to answer the self-funded or insured question for you, or at the very least, this information should be in the employee paperwork you filled out when you were first hired. As a last-ditch effort, the Employee Benefits Security Administration at the U.S. Department of Labor, https://www.dol.

gov/agencies/ebsa, should be able to get this information for you. You are paying for this health coverage—either out of your weekly paycheck or as a benefit allowed by the terms of your employment. Even though your employer is engaging it all on your behalf, you are entitled to know—and really should know—the specifics of the coverage you have through your work.

Here's an interesting story from LeAnn about health insurance and a testament to the wonderful way her husband's employer stepped up when it came to protecting her child when he needed insurance the most . . . and suddenly didn't seem to have it. It would be great if everyone had this kind of an outcome when they came to an insurance snafu.

My son was in the ICU, ready to have a stem cell transplant, and somehow, and I really still don't understand how this came to be, the hospital called to let us know that we were not covered for the stem cell harvesting. As you can imagine, this part of the procedure was vital, and we were indeed covered for every step of the procedure, just not this one part. Now, my son's life depended on him having this very costly procedure, and very quickly our options became pay out of pocket (not that we just happened to have thirty thou just lying around) or quit our jobs, go on Medicaid, run my son over to St. Jude's, and hope for the best.

This is when the company my husband works for really stepped up. We managed to get right up the ladder, to the CEO in fact, on this question of my husband's work health insurance, and within twenty-four hours we were told the company would pay for what my son needed. It was a blessing. It's amazing really how they came to our rescue like that, and we were so grateful.

But I know a positive outcome like this is a rare case. I hear the horror stories of too many families left broken financially over cancer care. They are either penalized by their insurance company along the way, or people have to uproot their families to find a facility that will take them, maybe they come to be treated in a hospital that's not the very best for their needs simply because the financial situation dictated they have to go where the insurance company says. Or insurance won't pay for simple things like a hotel stay when you have to go out of town for treatment or to clinical trials. There's so many places in the process where insurance coverage can break down or really be less than you need, and it's terrible.

And believe me, a hospital will tell you very quickly what exactly you owe.

❦

I'm heartened by the fact that many states require insurance companies to cover specific cancer screening and also provide free or low-cost screening and treatment programs for specific types of cancer. When it comes to cancer care, early detection is critical, a matter of life and death in many cases. The fact that insurance companies got with the program here simply means many more lives will be saved.

Prescreening, treatment, and the employer's rights are not the only concerns our laws and programs cover. For something particularly close to my heart, the **Women's Health and Cancer Rights Act (WHCRA)** is a federal law requiring health insurance companies whose policy covers mastectomy to also cover the reconstruction of the breast on which the mastectomy was performed, and surgery or reconstruction of the other breast to produce a symmetrical appearance. Prostheses and/or implants are also covered in many cases. The WHCRA also covers treatment for physical complications from mastectomy and will cover patients moving from one plan or another during this procedure. It does indeed seem breast cancer is no longer the taboo subject it was when my mother was first diagnosed in the late eighties; in the two programs above, both pre– and post–breast cancer concerns are covered.

Currently, certain states require insurance companies to cover routine costs of clinical trials. The **Patient Protection Affordable Care Act (ACA)** put extra onus on insurance companies not to deny or restrict costs for patients being considered for, or undergoing, trials. Simply prepping for participation in a clinical trial can be stressful, and having the ACA in place alleviates some of that stress.

Genetic Testing and Insurance

Recently, genetic testing is being considered both by the law and insurance companies. This is another step in the right direction, as far as I'm concerned.

As I wrote in chapter 1, I underwent a double mastectomy two years ago to greatly lessen my chances of getting breast cancer. While I didn't have any genetic mutation that conclusively related to a risk of breast cancer, I did have mutations that are currently of unknown significance, and they were the same ones my sister has. She, and my mother, developed breast cancer. While I know many people, doctors among them, are against what they consider such a drastic preventive measure, I am bound and determined to stick around for as long as I can. Genetic research is still in its infancy, but we are learning more all the time, and my mantra is, I want to find out all the information I can, even if we have yet to understand what it all means. As of this writing, scientists believe that approximately 5% of all cancers are from hereditary risks; we can all certainly understand why people might want to get tested for predispositions and DNA connections.

The flip side to this, of course, is that the results of genetic testing could be used against patients. Insurance companies could use it to decide whether to insure someone, splitting semantic hairs that a genetic marker could be considered a preexisting condition. These concerns, with more patients wanting testing and how to be sufficiently covered for them, as well as what an insurance company or even an employer could do with this information, have yet to be fully realized and legislated. But it is all coming and will be an important part of the insurance and healthcare question in no time, I feel.

Certain health insurance policies currently in place *do* cover genetic testing; Medicaid currently covers certain genetic testing in twenty-six different states. And through the **Genetic Information Non-Discrimination Act (GINA)**, patients are already protected in their workplace against those discriminations I mentioned, as well as HIPAA protecting against "genetic discrimination."

We have a long way to go as the field of genetic research grows, but rest assured, whatever health insurance you have, it will be affected in some way in the near future by scientific breakthroughs like genetic testing.

Legal Questions and Resources Beyond Insurance: What Legal Documents Should I Have in Place?

Whether you are nearing the end of your life due to a terminal illness or are facing a time where you will need assistance with managing your healthcare or finances, it is essential to make plans in advance to ensure your wishes are carried out in the event you become unable to make decisions on your own. You should gather all important records and documents in one place, and make sure your loved ones or caregiver are aware of where they are. The Cancer Legal Resource Center (www. Cancerlegalresources.org) offers a comprehensive list of documents that you should collect, which include:

- Your will, with the name and address of your attorney
- Power of attorney and advance directive
- Funeral or memorial instructions
- Financial information, including previous years' taxes, names of financial institutions you have accounts with, passwords, etc.

What Is an Advance Directive . . . And Do I Really Need One?

An advance directive protects your right to refuse medical treatment that you do not want, or to request treatment you do want in the event you lose the ability to make decisions yourself. There are typically two documents included in an advance directive: *a power of attorney for healthcare* and a *living will*. Each state will have specific requirements for these documents, but they generally cover the same information. You do not need a lawyer to prepare your advance directive, but you will need to follow your state's requirements with regards to having notarization, witnesses, and signatures.

Power of Attorney for Healthcare

If you are no longer able to make healthcare decisions for yourself, having a power of attorney for healthcare will allow whomever you have designated as your healthcare agent to make informed decisions on whether to accept, maintain, discontinue, or refuse any care, treatment, service, or procedure to maintain, diagnose, or treat a physical or mental condition on your behalf. While this form is fairly short and simply asks you to designate who will be your healthcare agent, it is extremely important to identify the right person.

Who should you ask to be your healthcare agent?

- Someone who understands your wishes and will be willing to accept the responsibility of making healthcare decisions for you

Who cannot be your healthcare agent (unless they are related to you):

- Your physician
- An employee of your healthcare provider
- An employee of a healthcare facility where you reside

Living Will:

A living will is a written, legal document that spells out medical treatments you would and would not want to be used to keep you alive, as well as other decisions such as pain management or organ donation. End-of-life care decisions that you should consider, and share your feelings about, can include:

- Whether you want your healthcare agent to be able to admit you to a nursing home or community-based residential facility for a short-term period to recuperate
- Whether you want life-sustaining procedures if doctors have determined you are in a persistent vegetative state
- Determining if and when you would want to be resuscitated by cardiopulmonary resuscitation (CPR) or by a device that delivers an electric shock to stimulate the heart
- Considering if, when, and for how long you would want to be placed on a mechanical ventilator
- Deciding if, when, and for how long you would want feeding tubes to be used

- Determining, if you were near the end of life, would you want infections to be treated aggressively or would you rather let infections run their course?
- Deciding what type(s) of comfort care (or palliative care) you would like used to keep you comfortable and manage pain, while abiding by your other treatment wishes; examples of this may include being allowed to die at home, getting pain medications, being fed ice chips to soothe dryness, and avoiding invasive tests or treatments

Once you have completed your advance directive, you need to talk to anyone who might be involved in your healthcare decision making. This includes family members, loved ones, and your healthcare providers. You want them to understand how you feel about medical treatment at the end of life. If you have a primary hospital that you go to for treatment, providing them with a copy of your advance directive can make communication easier when you are admitted.

As each state has its own format or requirements for these forms, several websites offer legal advice and help. I would urge you to speak with your personal attorney or visit a trusted website such as Caring Info (www. caringinfo.org), which offers free advance directive forms by state.

Job Status, For Patient and Caregiver

Fortunately, many federal and state laws are in place to protect patients. These run the gambit from malpractice to the ways someone might need to be protected in their job and their future. The Family and Medical Leave Act of 1993 (FMLA) came into law to help patients and their families better balance the demands of work against the possible time off from it that a patient or even a caregiver might need for cancer treatment. In the broadest sense, this seminal bit of legislation brings the idea of preserving the needs of the family vis-à-vis the patient, or even their caregiver's employment, to the forefront.

If you are no longer able to work or are trying to plan ahead in case you become unable to work, you may be looking for information about ways to replace your income. The Social Security Administration (SSA) offers options that may be able to help you, should you qualify. In addition, while many people need Social Security Disability Insurance (SSDI) benefits for the rest of their lives, some people recover enough to return to work. Ultimately, the Social Security Administration (SSA) would like people to reenter the workforce, so it provides incentives to make this transition easier. Information can be found at the Social Security Administration website, https://www.ssa.gov/disability/.

Your Checklist

I warned you this was a deep well of information, some of which you might not need right now. You may just want to skip to the resource page of this chapter, look up a specific law or agency that applies to your needs presently, and go forth. But I wanted to be as thorough as I could, knowing that I have only managed to dip my toe into the great big sea of information one needs to know or can further research about health insurance, legal matters, and cancer care. I'd like to leave you with this basic checklist to help yourself—details to take care of before, during, and after your care.

- Start keeping files. You need to gather together your health insurance paperwork—explanations of benefits (EOB), insurance contact numbers, as well as every piece of paper you get from your oncologist or any other healthcare professional you come to see. I mentioned this back at the beginning of the book, but if you think the paper and correspondence was building before, wait until you start putting your insurance papers into the mix! As with everything else in our lives, a whole bunch of computer programs are available to help you amass, contain, and easily access this information. So, do some research; you might stumble onto something that could really help you here.

- <u>Make sure all your healthcare providers are given all the pertinent information for your insurance at the outset</u>. Surely anyone who attends to you, from an oncologist to an acupuncturist, will first ask about the insurance you have. But make sure you have any information they could ask for at the ready. Also, if you have more than one insurance, let every single one of your healthcare professional's financial officers or managers know this as well.

- <u>Keep all insurance cards and prescription drug plan ID cards with you at all times</u>. Your healthcare professional is most likely going to ask to copy those ID cards. But it's a good idea to have these cards and plan information on you at all times anyway.

- <u>Make sure all your information, even something as seemingly mundane as a new email address, is current with all your providers</u>. Again, lots of what I advise here is seemingly obvious stuff. But when you are sick or your caregiver is running around stressed, the most basic details get forgotten. Keep all your basic information on you . . . and at the ready.

- <u>Read and reread any forms presented to you before signing</u>. This is where a caregiver or patient advocate can come in handy (which I cover in the next chapter). Having a second pair of eyes looking over your forms is always a good idea. Again, I am not playing the cynic here, but the cancer patient isn't always feeling their best and often glosses over papers put before them, simply wanting to escape an oncologist's office or treatment center before they throw up.

- Find out if you need pre-authorization for upcoming procedures or treatments . . . then make sure to get it. Usually this is explored by your healthcare provider's in-house staff. Rest assured, they are not going to be engaging in anything with you they won't be getting paid for, but you should also be checking for when you need pre-authorization and are going to get it. And remember: just because your insurance company pre-authorizes doesn't mean they guarantee payment. But confirming a pre-authorization in writing (email works too) will help you in the long run if you have to plead a case for payment.

- Get an itemized copy of the bill, for all treatments, procedures, and hospital stays. You may very well find some errors here; it happens more often than you think. Check dates and procedure numbers; look for any inconsistencies. Again, I'm not suggesting anyone is trying to skirt something by you intentionally, but people make mistakes. If you need your caregiver or an advocate with you to crunch the numbers and double-check wording, get them to help you.

- Get a copy of both the medical record and pharmacy ledger. The medical record is something you may very well be asking for, but a pharmacy ledger is not something patients always know exists. You are entitled to see an accounting of all the drugs you are given, as much as you are a breakdown of all procedures and treatments. Compare the medical record and that pharmacy ledger to your hospital's itemized bill. Sometimes patients find they are charged for procedures, drugs, or treatments that were ordered but never given to them. Again, get another pair of eyes if you need to, but check the paperwork that you are given and ask for.

- <u>If you know you might need to have one in place, negotiate your payment plan as soon as you can</u>. These days there are many options for payment, so research this from the provider of your services as much as from your insurance company . . . but do so as soon as you can. You need to get your payment plan in place and approved (again in writing) so there will be no confusion as to when and how much you pay on your bill. Treatment facility financial offices and collection agencies will go to the end of the earth trying to collect on an outstanding bill. In owing an amount that is past due you could get sued, adding compound interest to your balance, and all of this can badly affect your credit (and life) if you fail to pay a medical debt or prolong doing so for too long. It's best to get the how and when of your payments out of the way as early as you can, even if this means setting yourself on a payment plan for a prescribed period of time.

⟨◈⟩

Information is your first best weapon in the business of cancer care, as it is everywhere else. Knowing what kind of cancer you have, what treatment options are available, and what legal and financial recourses you have at your disposal is key. There will come reams of papers, lots of confusion and correspondence, and probably more phone calls needing to be made than you will ever want to make. You can make it all easier the more prepared you are and the more you research the business of your care.

Takeaways

- As with every other facet of your cancer care and concerns, you need to know the ins and outs of your health insurance as best you can.

- While certainly, federal changes in the law and each new administration will probably manage its own influence on U.S. healthcare—to your advantage or not—plenty of laws and legislation are in place to help the cancer patient understand and better use the insurance they have. Get to know these laws, statutes, and organizations as well as you know the intricacies of your insurance.

- Gather all your important documents, store them in a safe place, and make sure that your loved ones or caregivers know where to find them.

- Have an advance directive in place so that in case you are unable to make decisions on your own, your wishes are clearly outlined for your family and loved ones.

RESOURCES:

Patient Advocate Foundation (PAF), www.patientadvocate.org, 800-532-5274. In addition to the work they do with advocacy, they also offer a Co-Pay Relief Program which provides financial assistance to patients.

National Coalition for Cancer Survivorship, http://www.canceradvocacy.org/, 1-877-622-7937. The NCCS offers a list of online publications that explores the many types of health insurance and health coverage.

The Employee Benefits Security Administration at the U.S. Department of Labor, https://www.dol.gov/agencies/ebsa, can help you explore your employer's health plan particulars as well as answer any other questions concerning the law and your employee rights.

The Hill-Burton Program, available in all states except IN, NE, NV, RI, UT, or WY, offers reduced-cost healthcare services to patients who prove eligible. They can be reached by calling 1-800-638-0742.

The **National Breast and Cervical Cancer Early Detection Program (NBCCEDP)** runs an early detection program in conjunction with the Centers for Disease Control and Prevention (CDC). It helps low-income, the uninsured, and many other women the opportunity for breast and cervical cancer screening. Find them here: https://www.cdc.gov/cancer/nbccedp/index.htm.

The **Cancer Legal Resource Center Hotline** (866-THE-CLRC) matches cancer patients and survivors to volunteer attorneys. The CLRC can also provide information and resources on cancer-related legal issues and general legal advice www.Cancerlegalresources.org.

As mentioned previously, the **Leukemia and Lymphoma Society** is not only one of the best resources for patients with leukemia, lymphoma, or myeloma, it also offers assistance for services, treatments, transportation, and financial assistance for the insured's co-pays.

The **FMLA** can be reached here: (866) 487-9243 or (887) 889-5827 and at www.dol.gov/esa/whd/fmla.

Find out all your need to know about **HIPAA** (and plenty of other healthcare related laws) here:

https://www.hhs.gov/hipaa/for-individuals/guidance-materials-for-consumers/index.html.

National Hospice and Palliative Care Organization Caring Connections, 800-658-8898, www.caringinfo.org, offers financial advice for patients in hospice. It also offers free state-specific information on advance directives.

The Partnership for Prescription Assistance (PPA), 888-477-2669, www.pparx.org, is a free service that offers access to close to five hundred programs for free and low-cost drugs.

The Social Security Administration website: https://www.ssa.gov/disability/.

The **Employee Benefits Security Administration at the U.S. Department of Labor**, https://www.dol.gov/agencies/ebsa.

Chapter 7

So, You Are the Caregiver

As a trained nurse, my father was instrumental in taking care of my mother; he did more than any family member would normally be able to do. Rather late in her disease, when her cancer had metastasized, my mom needed to have chest tubes put in to drain the fluid that was building up around her lungs. Someone without my father's skills and training wouldn't have been able to drain these tubes on a daily basis. I know my mother was happy that he could handle it, but if Dad hadn't been able to, where would we have found help?

My father could have easily demurred. Although a nurse, he could have simply said that being my mother's nurse would have been too much for him, and we would all have understood. It is one thing to be the patient's spouse (or parent), but their caregiver as well? This is not a role everyone can easily take upon themselves, even if they have a professional skill set to do so. As LeAnn says, "The caregiver ends up really doing everything the patient does, short of taking the medicines and undergoing the treatments."

Remember, back when she was first diagnosed, I was recently out of my first semester of college. I had no clue how to care for someone, let alone my mom, sick with cancer. One of the big reasons I wanted to write this book is that, most of the time, the person who comes to care for a cancer patient, beyond that patient's professional healthcare team, will probably have little to no medical knowledge. Usually, it's just a family member, friend, lover, or parent thrust into the chaos of cancer care with no idea what to do, learning by the seat of their pants, quickly overwhelmed if not completely scared to death. Believe me, even if you do have some background or are like my dad with some knowledge of what to do, caring for someone like this is going to exhaust you. I can tell you that quite often my father and I were completely worn out caring for my mom, usually more emotionally than physically (and the emotional affects the physical, as you know). Your whole life changes so much when you have someone in our life who is chronically or seriously sick, be it from cancer or anything else. Fairly quickly, you can come to find that your life is not your own anymore. Time and again we lose ourselves in attending to the patient; I know I did. It's no small point and something I will get into in a bit here, but the caregiver certainly needs caring *in their own way.*

My family was blessed by the simple fact that we were close by, and I was able to make a job change that gave me more time with my mother. Plenty of caregivers do not live close to the patient, though. I have a friend whose dad got stricken with lung cancer. This older man lived in Texas at the time, and my friend —his daughter, was living in Europe. Best as I could, I coordinated her dad's care via email and phone calls, but my friend was not on hand. The strain on both my friend and her father being so far apart was enormous, but many cancer patients are in this position. Caregivers may be miles away, trying to facilitate care, finessing schedules, offering support, contacting family members and neighbors who have offered to help—and not able to be with their family member while they endure treatment. Luckily, even for those with on-hand caregivers, plenty of support mechanisms are in place to help.

Patient Advocates

The concept of patient advocacy has been around for quite a while, beginning in the U.S. in the latter part of the nineteenth century, and has been growing ever since. It is an area of specialization in healthcare concerned with *seeing to the rights and needs* of patients, survivors, and caregivers. The patient advocate may be an individual or an organization, often, though not always, concerned with one specific group of disorders.

The advocacy movement centers around the idea of healthcare professionals (the advocate) helping people find answers to their questions and concerns regarding treatment and the resources they may need. Back in the day, patients were often left in the dark over their care, not getting the help or answers they were seeking. The advocacy movement created a bridge for people to get the healthcare they were seeking and to get their questions answered about it.

Professionals, from healthcare workers to lawyers and social workers, helped out in these early stages by starting organizations like the American Society for Control of Cancer (the present-day American Cancer Society) and the National Foundation for Infantile Paralysis (known today as the March of Dimes). Fast forward into the 1970s, and advocacy was bolstered by the National Welfare Rights Organization's work in 1972. One of the first professional associations for advocacy began at this time as well, the Society for Healthcare Consumer Advocacy. This group helped see Sarah Lawrence College start a master's in health advocacy in 1980.

As we see presently, the complexity of the insurance industry and healthcare system can create plenty of obstacles for patient understanding and execution of their own care. The system is based on complex rules making care and treatment ever harder and harder for the layman to navigate and decipher. These days, advocates are needed more than ever, and certainly for those who do not have a personal network of friends and family around them. In the past few years, I have seen plenty of oncology departments and hospitals hiring their own advocates (also called navigators), offering this additional support to patients.

For the caregiver, the advocate can be an invaluable aid. You can seek out an advocate for a specific concern or for broad support. If you have questions about financial options for your treatment, the drugs that have been prescribed, finding psychological support, or even trying to coordinate transportation, there is an advocate for almost every concern. Advocates can also step in pre-treatment to discuss and lay out options during the phase when a patient and their caregiver are trying to determine what course of action is best for fitting all of what is about to happen into one's life. They can sit in on doctor-patient conferences or sit across from a patient at their home. They can lay out a mountain of paperwork and define each and every word.

Last, many advocates are trained in counseling. They can hold your hand (literally and figuratively) while you're sitting in the waiting room to see your doctor or when you are at home feeling alone and scared out of your mind.

Of course, with the good comes the bad. Many people are concerned that too many modern-day advocates are indeed being provided by a specific hospital, healthcare office, or even insurance company, and therefore that advocate might have a certain bias. This could well be true in some cases. As an example, advocates within insurance companies, often referred to as case managers, may reach out to members, offering education, perhaps about their diagnosis or specifics about their insurance benefits, and to help members navigate the system. While I don't want to be negative about the support these case managers may be able to provide to patients, part of their role is to coordinate care and treatment in the most efficient (and sometimes) cost-effective way for their companies. It is enough of a concern that some institutions lay out a code of ethics that provides power and autonomy to people in this role just to avoid this very issue.

My family has had experience with case managers, and while I've found them to be helpful in answering questions, I still feel more comfortable talking with a healthcare provider about treatment decisions and mapping out a plan for care. While some advocates are hired and work for specific companies, you can also find independent advocates who will work specifically for you. If you are looking to find and hire a personal advocate, you can find them at websites such as the *Advoconnetion Directory* or *Values Based Patient Advocates* (see both below in resources). These web portals provide patients with a list of private advocates and also provide a place for those advocates to register. As with the very best the Internet has brought us these days, with these websites, people connect as transparently as possible, and in this case, for an important cause.

Even the most knowledgeable, hands-on, sympathetic caregiver cannot do it all and cannot know everything there is to know. Advocates can indeed come in handy. They are skilled men and women who have worked in the field for a while, and they will be able to predict upcoming complications and can meet them and prepare you for them. For the patient with no caregiver, an advocate can prove an invaluable resource.

Supporting the Caregiver: Building a Personal Network

Living the "when it rains, it pours" axiom, the last years of my mother's life, when her cancer had metastasized and she was undergoing her clinical trial—and I was doing everything I could not to dwell on the facts and rationalize how long she had to live—I came to a crisis point at work.

Through a set of circumstances too complicated to get into (and nothing I even want to dwell on), it was becoming ever more apparent to me that when my big company was bought by an even bigger company, the company culture was going in a direction I didn't like anymore.

Before and during that first year of the last two years of my mother's life, I was living in Minneapolis with my family and working for a pharmaceutical company that I had been with six years at that point. Given the business I was in, where the specifics of cancer care were well known, when I presented the circumstances about my mom to my employers, they allowed me to work remotely. My husband and I made the decision to move back to Green Bay. I've come to regard my company being this flexible as another blessing, really.

But at the beginning of the second year of my mom's treatment, my company was bought out by a bigger company. The culture around my office began to change. My team was no longer being cultivated and appreciated in a way that made me comfortable. There were too many "cooks in the kitchen," and work that used to be challenging and fun for me was all too quickly becoming drudgery. Even working from home as I was, I could feel a sea change coming, and I wanted out. The writing was on the wall for me, and I decided to quit. My husband had been aware of how unhappy I was with the company of late and had been encouraging me to get out, but quick.

Was my mother's condition a factor for me leaving my job? Even now I'm not sure how much it played into my decision to get out when I did, but certainly, the timing was right. I had been thinking about what I would do if I had the opportunity to do whatever I wanted; I quickly admitted I'd love to open my own consulting business. A mere few months after quitting, I did indeed begin that business, one where I worked for the rest of my mother's life. Working for myself, though taxing the first year as I built my business, afforded me even more freedoms, and maybe even a good diversion from the constant reminder of what my mom was going through. (Time and again I will champion the idea of the caregiver needing their mental breaks.) Again, I recognize that I was blessed. Although I would trade any of this for my mother being alive right now, I am happy I slipped into a bigger caregiver role at that time, spelling my father even better than I had before.

Time was precious for us all during those last years of my mother's life; we all sensed that clock at our backs.

At this point I was as much another full-time caregiver to my mom as my dad. He was, and would always be, the primary caregiver, but I slipped in and out for both of them as I saw fit, or as they asked. Where Mom seemed to need a softer-edged emotional support for Dad, I was more of a cheerleader. (Mom didn't want anyone else cleaning her home, and only my father and I to ever cook or do the laundry. My mom used to say, "The last thing I want is to have someone else in the house when I feel terrible.")

There is an important point in all of this. When you come to be the secondary caretaker or just someone who comes in from time to time to give family members a break, if you can be a bit intuitive in seeing what each person needs, as befits their personality, you can really help. My father was the guy who cracked jokes all the time; he'd talk to anyone. His patients knew him as the nurse who'd distract them with a funny story so they'd never feel the IV going in. Giving forth of his big personality and deep charm was my father's way of dealing with life, especially so when trying to keep my mother's spirits high. For my father, I'd present dinner options or simply let him go out to run errands. He was, and still is, a social guy, and I knew he needed to get out of the house, be proactive, and take the actions he needed to deal with for himself. I was constantly facilitating what he needed with a "Yeah, Dad, go and do that; don't worry, I got this," approach, as that's what he most needed . . . and what I most wanted to give him.

For my mom, it was a softer approach, as I said. I'd sit with her and make lists—she loved her lists—of what needed to get done for the week. We'd sit in the house writing out thank-you cards, getting into the laundry, simply ticking things off her list that would bring her comfort. It really was all about easing her frustration level and getting to stuff that was most on her mind and that was becoming ever harder for her to attend to.

For both of my folks, I felt like a general contractor of cancer care. I saw to what they needed and facilitated those needs with my physical presence, and helped manage other people calling or coming over to lend their support. And believe me, managing these well-intentioned folks takes a lot of stress off the caregiver. Yes, by that point I had a lot of medical knowledge, and there were those times I did sit with my mother to go over some paperwork, but mainly it was more my personal and organizational skills I brought to the table.

No matter how private of a person you might be or you know the patient is, patient and caregiver can still avail themselves of friends and family looking to support you. It's not easy to take this help all the time. (I am sure there were as many times that my father was happy to see me as he maybe wanted to be alone; luckily, being as close as I was, I could usually read the times to stay away and the times to be there.) But even with the best intentions, friends and family wanting to do jobs for you the patient or you the caregiver occasionally come up with ideas that are not that helpful.

The first time my mother was diagnosed and going through her chemo treatments, friends and family would bring meals over to us . . . which was a nice gesture. Dad and I weren't really thinking about what we should be making for dinner, so having options was great. But when she was going through chemo, quite often my mom couldn't handle the smell of food, even things that didn't smell all that much or that my dad and I cooked. I can't tell you the number of times some scrumptious meal ended up in the freezer, or worse yet, wasted because we just couldn't eat it.

So how do you tap into the support around you and not have to feel like you are asking for help but are getting the help you need?

- Identify someone who is willing to coordinate support efforts for you. As the one dealing with the diagnosis, your focus can be on your health and recovery. If you are the primary caregiver, having a backup or additional support in place can also cut down on the number of times you have to personally answer the question: "What can I do to help?"
- Create a list of the things you might want some help with, and when people ask what they can do, you can either say, "Well, actually, there is something I could use a bit of help with," or provide them with that list. This could include driving a carpool, going to the grocery store, helping with laundry, watering your flowers, etc. As I say, my mom loved her lists, and people wanted to help. It was a perfect match.

This next point works for the patient with caregivers and for those patients whose potential helpers might not be so close by.

- Take advantage of social media if you are connected this way. Either the patient can update their Facebook page or create a Caring Bridge page, or their caregiver can. This is a great way to get in touch with people without having to see them in person. Certainly, there were many days my mom wanted to say hello or thank you to someone, but she wasn't getting out of bed.

This above point is not to be brushed over and, in fact, leads to something I want to expand on when it comes to caregivers looking for or being offered help.

Social Media as Part of Your Support Network

It's a weird and wobbly double-edged sword when somebody gets sick. Although the patient and their caregiver will very much want to reach out and ask for help—and there is often a large contingent of family, friends, coworkers, church friends, and neighbors who want to help—quite often the help doesn't come . . . or at least not exactly when and how it is needed. It's the unusual and unfortunate circumstance of a loved one getting sick. People usually don't know what to do or say . . . as much those suffering as those wanting to help. There is that hesitation, we've all seen it in action or have felt it ourselves, both sides not knowing how far they should go, trying so hard not to overstep in what they want to offer or what they might ask for. Yes, things have gotten better, but still, the asking for and the offering of help is a delicate dance, to say the least.

I have seen this in my own situation with my own family, even though, as I said, we were luckily a close-knit bunch; family and friends lived at most a half hour away. I was doing pretty well keeping everybody updated and handing out tasks if they asked. But I look back on this all now and think I should have used more of what was available at the time during the last few years of my mom's life, specifically to keep family, friends, and people who wanted to help us better informed. Any awkwardness or confusion could have been easily brushed aside had I gotten connected via social media.

I'm specifically thinking of the **Caring Bridge** website, but you can use any social media portal you like. Sites like **ShareTheCare.org** also provide information and resources on how to organize a group for caregiving help. (I list more of them at the end of this chapter, as I do in the big resource page at the end of this book.)

My family was never on Facebook, and we didn't sign up when my mother got sick. But I do understand the need to update people via the web, so any way you wish to do it, be it Caring Bridge, Twitter, Facebook—have at it, I say. If you are interested in sharing information with others (remember, it's always your choice), posting updates not only makes it possible for people to read about what's going on but can also clue them into what you might need if they do indeed want to reach out. I can't tell you the number of times I'd hear somebody ask, "What can I do? Just ask, and I will be there." Or somebody simply assuming we could use a meal or a ride, when at that particular time these offers, while all wonderful and heartfelt, weren't what we needed most. And sometimes, quite frankly, the caregiver doesn't want to get on the phone and start to go over, yet again, what the latest on the cancer patient is. It can be exhausting talking about the details of the illness over and over again. Simply being able to update almost everyone at once could be a relief.

I often wonder if things might have been easier if we had used some sort of social media. We were in constant contact with friends and family through phone calls, and my dad went to church every Sunday, so he was relating the latest news about my mom to his friends there. But I see now that a website like Caring Bridge would have been helpful, specifically in keeping with the way we like to deal with our personal business. Not that I am trying to sell you on this website, it's just that in the case of Caring Bridge you can put as much or as little of your story out to the people with whom you want to connect. It is a site (and again there are others just like it) made specifically for this purpose.

The wonderful thing about social media is, both parties can post as much or as little of their information as they care to. Many patients share a lot of information, and for some I know it is cathartic to write about their daily trials and treatments. Others want to share only the basic facts, as they don't have the energy or desire to belabor the point of what they are living through. Those friends and family who want to help or at least be kept up to date on a cancer patient's condition can read as much, or again, as little as they want. It can also provide a place where words of support and comfort, or thoughts and prayers, can be shared. All the phone calls and cards and letters my mom received were wonderful, but she found them to be exhausting as well. She felt that if someone called, she should answer, and every card deserved a written response or a thank you. The use of social media could have made things easier for her.

Taking Care of Yourself

As LeAnn is quick to point out, and I wholeheartedly agree, the caregiver usually finds themselves doing everything the patient does, save undergoing treatment and suffering through the actual physical and mental aspects of the cancer. LeAnn and her husband with their son Cameron, my dad and I with my mom: anyone who is there on a regular basis attending to the patient truly feels the weight of the world on their shoulders at times. Therefore, that warning I began this chapter with—that the caregiver can so easily lose themselves in caring for a patient—is not something you should take lightly. Making sure medicines are given on a specific schedule, finding food or beverages that appeal to your loved one, fluffing pillows, updating their Netflix queue, parking the car at the hospital, and being present so intently can easily come to exhaust you. You might also find you're beset with terrible guilt when you want to do anything for yourself.

But your life needs to go on. No person you care for wants their illness to rob you of your life! My mom would often remind us that we needed to take care of ourselves.

So how do you protect yourself? How does the caregiver take care to make sure they get care, beyond having another person on hand to take over or give them a break occasionally?

First and foremost, you must keep yourself healthy. Yes, the person you are caring for might not ever truly be in the mood to eat, and when they do it could be they can only handle certain smells or tastes. I already told you about the many times my dad and I had to throw out food simply because my mother couldn't stand the smell. But you have to eat, and you have to eat well. Catching a burger at a drive-thru is all right in a pinch, but without regular good nutrition you are going to get sick, or at the least, not be at your best.

Along these same lines, of course, you need to get rest—not just a good eight hours (or whatever amount you are used to getting that gets you to function) but breaks from caregiving. On watch, while the patient sleeps will not bring you the most restful sleep, even if you do get to sleep during those times. Get a good amount of sleep, and as much in your own bed as possible.

Basic stuff? Certainly. Important? Absolutely.

Third, live your life. If there are things you need to attend to, you must make time for them. If you have activities that you engage in on a regular basis that bring you pleasure, that exercise your mind, body, and brain, do not stop doing them. As I mentioned, you might feel the initial pangs of guilt or selfishness creeping in considering your seemingly trivial needs when the person you are caring for is suffering, but work to get over it. You need to live your life.

Yes, it's all well and good me suggesting that you attend to the above, trying to impress upon you to put yourself first sometimes, but I know it's not so easy when you are the primary caregiver for the patient. You need to take care of yourself, because if you don't, at the very least, you won't be able to take care of the patient.

Last, you need to acquiesce to that which you cannot do. Everyone has talents as much as they do limitations, even the most highly skilled people. Like I say, my dad and I were blessed both by the skills we possessed that we could use and from our support system; we didn't face what we couldn't do all that often. When I think back to what I personally could not do, I remember near the end, when my mother and I both knew how long she had left. We never discussed it. In her mind, this was not a discussion to have with me, her daughter. She wanted to spare me the pain of this conversation. You must recognize your limitations as a caregiver and realize when you need to take a step back. This is why secondary caregivers, building a network, and/or enlisting an advocate can be so helpful.

Parent Caregiver

Being a parent caregiver is not a situation any of us wants to consider, certainly. But being caregivers to a child with cancer is a wholly unique situation. I am blessed to have a friend like LeAnn, because she is such a warm and wonderful person. We can truly learn from her experience here, as difficult as it might be to consider. I will let LeAnn give you her viewpoint about parent as caregiver.

I think for everyone there is a fight-or-flight response, whether patient or caregiver, suddenly you are in a circumstance that could easily, and so often does, undermine all relationships. As a caregiver you need to find peace, best you can during these times; the chronic stress management you are trying to deal with is off the charts. For the parent of a child diagnosed with cancer, I can report things definitely became trying in so many different ways. For instance, how do you tell your other child about what his brother is going through and what to expect? We have an older son and we needed to be mindful of his emotions, of how he was coming to handle his younger brother being sick as much as we had to care for Cameron. Then how do you tell your sick child that you are holding him down for his own good when he's about to undergo some painful procedure? How do you basically watch as the person you are supposed to protect the most in the world is suffering through something you are pretty much powerless against?

I remember when I wasn't exactly getting the response I wanted from Cameron's doctor. We certainly enjoyed a love/hate relationship during Cameron's care, though I'm happy to say we are good friends now. He's a really great guy, a wonderful doctor. But at this one particular time my brain was either on overload or he wasn't explaining himself good enough, and I said to him: "You might be the doctor here, but I am the mother. I'm the one with the MBA when it comes to this kid. Sorry, but my knowledge here surpasses yours, so you have to make me understand what you are saying."

❦

Taking care of a cancer patient, as the primary caregiver, presents a set of circumstances as well as challenges unique to most people's experience. Some recommendations that can help you manage the stressors you are facing:

- Tap into support from social workers, counselors, nurses, psychologists, and doctors.
- Lean on family members or friends, talking with them or letting them help with household needs.
- Continue to take care of yourself. Learn ways to reduce anxiety or tension, such as exercising, listening to music, or keeping a journal.
- Find strength in religious beliefs or spiritual practices.

Some additional recommendations specifically for parents who are caregivers:

- Find a way to take control of decisions involving your child as much as possible.
- Find support groups or other opportunities that will let you talk with other parents of children with cancer.

I just hope some of the information above makes your way easier, no matter where it is you happen to land in the equation. Remember, your help is always appreciated, even if you don't exactly always know what's best to offer or say.

Takeaways

- The patient's caregiver, be they family member, spouse, or friend, often plays a big role in the patient's care.
- Patient advocacy is a viable source for caregivers and patients alike.
- Building and maintaining a care network can be essential, and many tools are available—social media among them—to help the caregiver and patient keep in touch with those people who want to help.
- A caregiver must be careful to take care of themselves when attending to the cancer patient. It is all too easy for someone to get lost in

the day-to-day of attending a sick person and not see what they, themselves, might need.

RESOURCES:

The American Cancer Society's **Caregivers and Family** website, https://www.cancer.org/treatment/caregivers.html, 800-277-2345, is a full resource for what caregivers can come to expect.

The Caregiver Action Network, https://www.cancersupportcommunity.org/caregivers, is a specific web portal for caregivers, championing their specific needs.

The Cancer Net, https://www.cancer.net/coping-with-cancer/caring-loved-one, is designed for caregivers exclusively.

Share the Caregiving Inc., https://sharethecare.org/, is a not-for-profit program set up for the "quality of life" of caregivers.

Caring Bridge Network, https://www.caringbridge.org, is a social network specially designed for cancer patients and their personal network of caregivers, friends, and family.

Advocacy

Patient Advocate Foundation (PAF), www.patientadvocate.org, 800-532-5274, offers assistance to both insured and uninsured patients, helping in coordinating benefits and managing of cases.

The AdvoConnection Directory, https://advoconnection.com/, is a large resource where patients and private advocates can connect.

Values Based Patient Advocates, https://valuesbasedpa.com/, (703) 222-1300, lists advocates who are 100% unbiased.

Chapter 8

End-of-Life Decisions

Those last few days in the hospital, all of us were fully aware of where Mom's health was at; we all knew that she was most likely going to die in a matter of days. I remember needing to hear my mother say that she was done fighting and ready to let go. None of us wanted to verbalize what was happening, but what made the difference to me—more than knowing how far her cancer had spread, knowing that my parents had dealt with their lawyer and my mom's will just a week before, knowing that her body was shutting down, knowing that Mom's oncologist had told her there was nothing else to try—was hearing my mother say that she was done with all the treatments and the trying. As I sat next to her, I thought she was sleeping until she opened her eyes and said to me: "I'm ready to go."

This was all I needed. When we took her from the hospital back to my parents' home, we called in hospice; I knew we were doing exactly what my mother wanted.

Even though my mother did die of cancer that spread through her body, we came late to hospice. We took my mother from the hospital on a Monday, knowing all along that she wanted to die at home. Hospice services came to my parents' home that very day, worked at the house Tuesday and Wednesday, and my mother passed three a.m. that Thursday morning.

I realize most people don't come to hospice like this. In many cases, hospice care comes into the patient's home (statistics currently show that

70 percent of hospice care takes place in a patient's home) or a patient is admitted into a hospice facility weeks, even months before they die. Hospice care is also available in special units in hospitals and nursing homes. I'll let Joyce weigh in here about the differences between going to a facility and having hospice come into your home.

There is an important distinction to be made between hospice care being provided at home and the kind of hospice where a patient is admitted to a facility that provides hospice care. Certainly, the facility care is not for everyone, not a choice appropriate for a good percentage of patients and their families (as Deb says above, more hospice occurs in the home than in a facility), but at other times it is exactly the kind of palliative care (medical care for people with serious illnesses) some people need if complex care and pain management is required.

In some cases, a cancer patient needs complex pain medication management that could be beyond the scope of what hospice can offer in their home. Conversely, some patients want to remain in their home—a safe and familiar environment where they can enjoy their family, and they can take part in the care during this time.

Both types of hospice can work just fine, and it is just up to the patient and their caregivers to decide which suits them specifically. Talking with the medical team and understanding how either option would work is important.

⚜

What happened with my mom was a rare case in how little actual time we needed hospice. Believe me, I know the very word "hospice" sends shivers down the spine, for even those people blessed enough never to have had anyone in their family, even distant relatives, avail themselves of this end-of-life care. But for many, hospice is a fact of life, and as ever, I want you to get the facts straight.

The subject of hospice care for a cancer patient is typically introduced by a patient's oncologist when the expectation is that the patient is likely to survive less than six months. Of course, this time frame varies for different reasons (which I will explore in a bit), as nobody, least of all a doctor, truly knows when a patient is going to die. In my mother's case, she had no other treatment options left, her lungs were pretty much compromised with chest tubes having to be implanted in her, and her heart wouldn't have withstood any more treatment had any more been offered to her. It's when treatment options are exhausted like this, as my mother's doctor told her they were, that the oncologist, concerned about making their patient as comfortable as possible, will make a recommendation for hospice.

Just six months before my mother died, she had undergone a procedure called a thoracostomy; those chest tubes were put in to drain fluid around her lungs. She also had a procedure called pleurodesis, in which medication was put in through those chest tubes to try and reduce/eliminate fluid accumulation. While Dad was draining those tubes and Mom was still living life in her fashion, we could all see the end coming. My mother's lungs and heart were just too weak to withstand any more procedures, and she was in lots of pain; it was extremely difficult to see her suffering.

Was it the wisest choice for my mom to have gone through those last procedures, to have her doctor even recommend them? Should her oncologist have pushed for hospice at that six-month mark? Should he have dissuaded my mother from those last-ditch effort procedures? Looking back with hindsight, I still can't answer these questions definitively. Although, as I said at the outset here, maybe if we had brought hospice in at the time my mother went through that round of her last and debilitating treatments, her quality of life might have been better . . . she did have a terrible last few months. It's not that I think bringing hospice in earlier would have prolonged her life, I just see now that she might have been more comfortable when those last treatments she had were ineffective anyway.

The thing was, the oncologist knew that my mother was always saying: "next." She was predisposed always to be focusing on another treatment, always looking for options. She was a realist; she never even considered alternate treatments. She was always grounded in what was safely and scientifically available for her cancer. But my mother didn't want to leave any stone unturned in her fight to live her life to the fullest. It's because of this that I feel Mom's oncologist read her correctly; he knew my mother would not be content unless she tried whatever else was out there. Sure, hospice was looming on the horizon, and like me, the doctor didn't want to give up hope or maybe even face the inevitable. But even if hospice had been mentioned that half a year before she died, I'm not sure my mother would have wanted things any other way than the way they played out.

I will say that hospice was wonderful, even for those few short days we had them. In fact, my father called hospice at four thirty a.m. that Thursday morning, just after my mom died. A hospice nurse was at the house in less than half an hour. She called the coroner and the funeral home, and within two hours my mother's body was removed from the house. Within twenty-four hours my mom's hospital bed was removed as well. It was a blessing for us all that these details were taken care of so efficiently.

The interesting thing about hospice is that, although a whole host of professionals is on hand ready to attend the dying patient, it's really up to the patient and their family to determine how exactly they want hospice to attend them. For all intents and purposes, hospice follows your lead.

Remember what Joyce said, "It is just up to the patient and their caregivers to decide which suits them specifically." This is the basis of how hospice is best engaged.

In some cases, the caregiver/patient will want hospice to only provide an in-house nurse to manage the more involved medical procedures the dying patient might need. Other times, hospice nurses and volunteers provide more round-the-clock care. In some instances, specific care protocols need to be maintained, and at other times, a patient simply needs a consistent round of medicine to be administered to them to constantly keep their pain at bay. In fact, much of what hospice does, seeing as they are quite often hired to make the dying as comfortable as possible, is administer professional pain management—a very real concern for those dying of a life-threatening illness.

We should also consider that beyond attending to the sick and dying, hospice can provide invaluable resources to the caregivers and family of the patient. Many hospice companies and facilities provide grief counselors. Plenty have access to further resources that the survivors can avail themselves of. Beyond the work they do by reaching and supporting specific patients, hospice organizations often make resources available to churches and community centers, where you can find information for your end-of-life care questions and concerns.

There are so many ways to engage hospice, and a wide variety of services they can provide, even if the result of their care is always the same.

Here are some things to consider when choosing which hospice is right for your specific needs.

- *Does the hospice service you are engaging or considering have references you can check?* A recommendation from your oncologist, from a facility caring for you, or even a family who has recently used hospice could be all the vetting you need to determine if one hospice fits your needs over another. Again, the more time you have in considering hospice, the more time you will have to consider which hospice is best for you or your loved one.

- *How long has the hospice been in business?* There are perfectly competent hospice companies that have only been open for a few years. But with any business, the more years a provider has been doing the specific job they do, especially in a competitive field, might speak to how competent they are.

- *Is the hospice you chose Medicare certified?* I'll get into paying for hospice in a minute. A hospice being Medicare certified is of special concern for the patient who is a Medicare beneficiary.

- *Is the hospice accredited or state licensed?* Although it is not required that a hospice need be accredited to operate, it is good to know that an accredited hospice has been vetted by a third party.

- *What are this particular hospice's limits on treatment?* Is this hospice able to meet your specific needs? Some hospice services have grief counselors on hand to help the families of loved ones in hospice. As I explained, the hospice we hired made calls to the funeral home for us and took my mother's body out of the house. Some hospices also provide respite care for caregivers.

- Especially pertinent when hospice is coming to a private home: *What is the hospice's response times, and where are they located in relationship to where the patient lives?* As I explained, the hospice that attended my mother was faster than I could have ever dreamed coming to our house during those early morning hours when my mother died. As a side note, the hospice we used also checked up on my dad for a full year after my mom died.

Paying for Hospice

Most people who use hospice care are elderly. This means quite a few of the hospice population are entitled to Medicare Hospice Benefit and Medicaid (veterans are covered as well). These statistics are skewed, though, when we consider cancer patients who come to use hospice; unfortunately, cancer can come to any person at any age.

So how does somebody not yet over sixty-five or a veteran pay for hospice?

Many private insurance companies do provide some allowance for a portion of the cost of hospice care. As already noted, there are a wide variety of insurance companies out there, as well as types of insurance, each with their own set of qualifications and criteria. You'd have to check in with your insurance on how or if you are covered for hospice.

If you do not have insurance coverage and cannot otherwise afford hospice, sometimes the cost of the service is provided by donations and grants, gifts and other programs via a community or other outreach program.

Pediatric Hospice

While hospice care is a wonderful resource, in many cases it is still targeted toward caring for older people, not children. I'm going to let LeAnn share her story on what she experienced with Cameron and pediatric hospice, which highlights the need to continue to advocate for what you need.

I'm not sure how it is in a big city like New York, but I can tell you with where we live in North Carolina, certainly not a remote area by any means but again not a big city, there is no pediatric hospice. Hospice is typically set up for eighty-year-olds, not eight-year-olds. When the doctor came in to tell us basically there was nothing else they could do for Cameron, we were really at a loss.

There was no facility, no patient advocacy, no hospice program for kids dying of cancer. We had someone come out to our house, but after just a little while I had them just go; I could do better for Cameron than they ever could.

Surely, this was a few years ago, and God knows I have been to conferences and spoken on this issue plenty, but at the time, there was nothing in place for end-of-life care for a child. Really, you haven't experienced the terrible end of things until you are going with your husband to pick out a coffin for your child while he is still living. This is something we did about six months before Cameron died.

⊙≫≪

Yes, there should have been more resources available for LeAnn and Cameron. But just as our knowledge of cancer has evolved, and newer and better treatments have been discovered, what we have available for hospice, especially for children, has improved. The National Hospice and Palliative Care Organization (NHPCO.org) has established a pediatric advisory council which is focused on improving access to hospice and palliative care for children and their families —both within the U.S. as well as internationally. Great resources available at the NHPCO website, and others such as GetPalliativeCare.org, allow you to search for providers that have the experience in caring for children with serious illness.

The DNR

Do not resuscitate (DNR) is a legal order written either in the hospital or on a legal form to withhold resuscitation (CPR) or life support in respect of the wishes of a patient in case their heart were to stop or they were to stop breathing. Although not hospice specific, I feel the DNR is certainly part of the overall fabric of what we are discussing in this chapter. The DNR request is usually made by the patient or healthcare power of attorney, put in place through a physician order, and allows the medical teams taking care of the patient to respect their wishes. A DNR does not affect any treatment other than that which would require intubation or CPR. Patients who are DNR can continue to get chemotherapy, antibiotics, dialysis, or any other appropriate treatments.

You don't need to have an advance directive or living will to have do not resuscitate (DNR) and do not intubate (DNI) orders. You can make your preferences known to your physician, who can write the orders and put them in your medical record.

If you have a living will, however, be sure to mention in it whether you have a DNR or DNI order on file.

As I have mentioned plenty of times in my story, and not to inject any religious notion into the text, I do believe there are moments when we are blessed in life. Through the kindness of strangers, a seeming accidental occurrence, or a loved one proving to you, once again, how much you mean to them, time and again we all experience these moments when we need to take a step back and say, "Yeah, I am blessed!" This is how I feel, even with the few short days that we had hospice for my mother. We are blessed that there is a community of professionals attending people who are coming to the end of their life (and I sure hope we will see a further reaching and more complete pediatric hospice, as LeAnn says), and through the hospice worker's caring and professionalism, they bring grace and dignity to a most trying time.

Takeaways

- Start considering and even vetting hospice companies as early as you can.
- Hospice works to your specifications and can provide a wide variety of services.
- There are various ways you can pay for hospice, some you might even be covered for presently with the insurance you have.
- Legal documents like a DNR can also assure end-of-life decisions are carried out to the letter.

RESOURCES:

National Hospice and Palliative Care Organization Caring Connections, 800-658-8898, http://www.caringinfo.org/i4a/pages/index.cfm?pageid=1, is a deep well resource for people coming to end-of-life decisions.

The **American Hospice Foundation (AHF)**, https://americanhospice.org/, closed in June 2014, but you will still find here a wealth of information about hospice.

The **National Cancer Institute**, https://www.cancer.gov/about-cancer/advanced-cancer/care-choices/care-fact-sheet, webpage for end-of-life care.

The **American Cancer Society**, https://www.cancer.org/treatment/end-of-life-care/nearing-the-end-of-life.html, same page as above.

The **National Association for Home Care & Hospice (NAHC)**, https://www.nahc.org/, webpage for the trade association of resources, education, and advocacy for hospice and the people who need it.

Caring Connections of the National Hospice and Palliative Care Organization, http://www.caringinfo.org/i4a/pages/index.cfm?pageid=3289, 800-658-8898. Patients and caregivers can find a downloadable PDF applicable for each U.S. state cancer care and hospice.

Chapter 9

How to Survive Surviving Cancer

So, I have given you a rundown on hospice, mentioned the DNR, and expounded on specific end-of-life decisions that I truly hope you don't have to come to. It's a necessary subject to cover in a book about cancer, but I'd much rather be here, at this last chapter, presenting this positive, empowering wrap-up. If you are a survivor of cancer, someone who is caring for a survivor, someone who has survived a spouse, child, or friend who succumbed to cancer, or even if you are in the middle of treatment and seeing some positive results, I welcome you here and to a continued healthy life.

Survivorship is certainly of a different order these days than it was way back when my mother was first diagnosed or even when the dermatologist found my melanoma. In fact, advances in medicine and science have blown wide open the whole idea of survivorship. Back when my mother was first diagnosed, surviving cancer was simply about the specific steps of a patient who was diagnosed, then treated (which could have as much meant surgery as chemo, and usually always chemo); a patient lost their hair, threw up a lot, and if lucky, saw their cancer go into remission. As I have described, most of us who ended up cancer free, by treatment or surgery, survived to enjoy seeing our checkups stretch from a six-month frequency to a year. If one got to the five-year mark, they pretty much thought they were on the home stretch to living without cancer.

But advances in science have led to better and earlier detection, more effective treatments, networking for patient support, preventive care and genetic testing that is seeing a significant decrease in cancer taking hold or even beginning in some cases. There are even instances where cancer simply becomes a chronic condition. I am specifically thinking here of certain chronic leukemia patients taking a pill every day to keep their cancer at bay and simply going on with their lives. And look at Jimmy Carter—his cancer spread to his brain, but because of some aggressive immunotherapy called pembrolizumab, the ex-president shows no sign of cancer as of this writing; Valerie Harper as well is living with her brain cancer. Both of these people, as well as so many others, would have died from their advanced stages of cancer only a few years ago. Those of us who are surviving are doing so for better and longer, and for some cancer is indeed a condition that can be maintained.

Most of what we talk about when we ponder the changes of cancer survivorship has occurred within the past five years. This past half decade has seen such blistering fast advances in technology and scientific research, we can hardly keep up. This is all positive, of course; more people living on after their cancer treatments is a wonderful result gained from medical advances. It leaves a survivor (and their caregivers) a chance to see a nice, long life ahead of them while wondering what the heck they have just been through and where exactly they are going.

A good problem to have!

Cancer survivors should consider a survivorship plan.

Presently with cancer patients seeing a better quality of life before, during, and after their treatments; less invasive procedures and better drugs being used; higher survivorship rates overall; early detection increasing a patient's chances and quality of life, suddenly we face other concerns, those we simply did not have before. People are living on after receiving treatments that didn't exist a few years ago.

As important as it was to understand your diagnosis and your treatment options, equally important is to talk with your doctor about a survivorship plan. Discuss what you might expect when your treatment is over, what kind of lingering changes, either mental or physical, you might expect. What resources are available to help you through this transition phase from active treatment to survivorship?

The Mental

Recently I took my son to the dentist. He was not keeping up with his dental hygiene, as kids his age are wont to do. The way I look at this mom job I have, it's one of my job requirements to stay on my son and his brothers about this kind of stuff. The hygienist at our dentist's office warned my son that once gum disease sets in, even if it is taken care of, the patient always has it. This was when the hygienist offered an analogy. He said, "It's just like when somebody has cancer; that person always has cancer, even if it goes into remission." You can imagine my son rolling his eyes, knowing what was coming from me.

I was duty bound to explain to the hygienist that, although there are cancer patients who do indeed go into remission only to present with cancer later, patients can get cured of cancer.

I come to this section from the perspective that from my mom's first diagnosis, surgery, and treatment, we all considered her cured of breast cancer the first time she presented with it. There was no more cancer in her body. That my mother presented with breast cancer again fourteen years later, underwent treatment, and had it recur two years later, when it took her life, doesn't make her any less a survivor in that near decade and a half she was cancer free.

It's also true that oncologists these days are more confident in declaring patients cured because certain types of cancer, if caught early, are highly unlikely to show up again. Take my melanoma. It was cut out of me. Though I continue to go back to have regular checkups, I have never looked back thinking I was only in remission from it; I am cured.

Overall, it is a mind-set, I understand. There are whole legions of cancer patients who have not presented with a tumor in decades, who still view their survivorship the way that hygienist does; they are living with cancer and will always have it even if it never presents again. An equal number of folks feel they are cured of their cancer. Sure, whichever camp you are in, you are aware of what happened in your past, and you are most likely more proactive about your health than the average person.

Phil has an interesting perspective on the mental stress from survivors over being cancer free for a long period of time.

When a patient survives cancer, there is joy, but this comes along with a healthy dose of anxiety. In my experience, the anxiety is related to concern the cancer could return as well as concern there will be long-term side effects associated with treatment. For many people, these anxieties greatly blunt their happiness, and these concerns come up frequently—even daily despite good general health. For others, it is less of an issue day to day but flares as a follow-up appointment approaches on the calendar or whenever an ache or pain develops. That honeymoon period especially brings with it a terrible anticipation in some people that the longer they are cancer free that the next time they go in for a test or scan, the ticking time bomb will catch up with them.

I always make sure to tell patients to call me when they are really starting to get nervous, when the stress of what's coming gets too much. Oftentimes, just telling a patient that what they are feeling is normal, assuring them that so many patients feel the same way, makes their fear go away. In the extreme cases, I'd simply assure a patient that if they wanted to move their appointment time up, reschedule for an earlier screening, I was perfectly happy to do this. This kind of plays back on the point I made back in the beginning, of making sure you find a doctor you can communicate with. In a case like this, you might be communicating with him or her for many years after your treatment, during your survivorship, in fact.

This is all to say that surviving cancer is not easy; not easy to accept a diagnosis of cancer, and then endure its treatment. But the difficulty does not end with what appears to be successful treatment. In fact, we do not know if someone is cured of cancer until they die of other causes. That uncertainly makes survivorship especially demanding and is bound to alter one's outlook on life.

The Physical

The immediate physical effects of cancer and its treatment are known all too well to patients as well as caregivers; in most cases, these are called the side effects. Certain of these symptoms are specific to whatever kind of cancer or treatment one endures; other side effects seem to be more common across the board. I'm thinking mainly of nausea and fatigue here. But for some survivors of cancer, long-term physical considerations, impairments, and discomforts can be multitudinous, beyond just temporary discomforts and pain.

I'll use myself as an example. I had my double mastectomy and reconstruction surgery. This kind of surgery is becoming more common, not just for women presenting with a tumor but for those many women, like me, looking to avoid a heightened risk. For women undergoing these procedures, the long-term physical effects are evident, like the reality that breastfeeding children, if ever a consideration, now cannot be. Regardless of how, or if, the patient deals with prosthetics and reconstruction, your body image is forever altered.

With mastectomies, body image is one of the biggest considerations to the procedure, I feel. Some potential long-term complications/medical concerns (i.e., issues with implants) may come up as well. How you have come to see yourself for so many years and seeing yourself in a wholly new way (even though you might indeed survive cancer!) can leave you feeling shaken.

Other treatments can have both mental and physical implications. Women undergoing a hysterectomy from cancer or its treatment, while having less *outward* body image issues, often have a whole host of internal issues. Many women report feeling barren after a hysterectomy, even if they are well beyond the age of childbearing; and certainly the results of a hysterectomy can lead to some physical changes for a woman via hormone changes and menopause.

There are also those patients who undergo other kinds of significant cancer surgery and treatment that leave them needing to catheterize themselves on a regular basis or those who have to use a colostomy bag post-treatment. Surely, advances in science have made these physical concerns easier to negotiate—relatively speaking—but if you are the patient left with these extreme personal changes in your life, these can be unfavorable things to deal with.

There's also a symptom called *chemo brain* that often burdens a patient after chemo treatments. Described best as a brain fog, cancer patients often find their memory failing, some cognitive skills lessened, and a general fuzziness in their head after treatment. Usually, chemo brain fades the longer one is away from their chemo treatment, and after time usually dissipates completely. But this is a real physical ailment many patients experience.

Some patients also complain about and must live with long-term or even lifetime neuropathy—a damage or disruption to their nerves after various cancer treatments. Patients may present with tingling at the tips of their fingers or toes, a lessening in the strength of their hands, etc. Neuropathy can become a difficult physical problem.

Certainly, there are plenty of short-term as well as lifelong side effects for the removal of organs, and especially for patients undergoing amputation to keep their cancer from spreading (which is possible for some bone cancers).

The Financial

The financial burden of tests, long-term procedures, treatments, and purchasing drugs—even when one has a prescription plan—leaves plenty of cancer patients strapped for cash. Some people even have to declare bankruptcy as they become cancer free. A good percentage of cancer patients miss so much work undergoing treatment or must quit their jobs completely that there is often little or no money coming in during the ordeal of cancer treatment, but certainly a lot goes out.

Then there are those who need to continue to take specific medicines for a long time after their treatment, maybe for the rest of their lives. Other people will need to buy health supplies they have never had to buy before, after specific treatments or procedures.

As I wrote about in the insurance section, a person can't currently be denied insurance for a preexisting cancer diagnosis. But insurance companies now seem to be exacting fees from their clients with preexisting conditions with some very creative charges.

Simply put, a whole host of financial concerns come with survivorship. I recommend that you revisit the earlier discussion on insurance and resources available to help with the financial aspects of cancer treatment. If you are having trouble managing all your expenses, you may want to contact a financial counselor to help you plan a budget. You can also look online to find nonprofit consumer credit counseling services in your area.

Fertility

A highly specific set of survivor concerns come into play for mothers-to-be, women contemplating pregnancy, men who want to eventually father a child, and even for the couple who have had kids already.

When I was diagnosed with melanoma, soon after, I found out that I was pregnant (although I would subsequently miscarry). My doctor later told me that had he known I was going to present with cancer, he would have seriously cautioned me about trying to get pregnant. The way my cancer treatment played out, I needed no chemo, I had surgery, and it never returned. But the risks to a fetus are often high when the mother is undergoing treatment for cancer; not to mention the risk of difficulties conceiving for that woman down the line, after she has received these kinds of therapies.

Chemotherapy works by attacking cells that are rapidly dividing. This is how and why it gets cancer cells, but at the same time, this is why a cancer patient's hair falls out, since hair follicles constantly divide. Sperm and egg cells are also affected by chemo treatment. For women, treatments can put them into menopause, with no guarantee about the long-term impact on fertility. If a woman is able to conceive after treatment, and hoping to breastfeed, she may not have this option after treatment for breast cancer. For men, testicular cancer or even other types of cancer and the treatments used can leave him sterile. This topic should come up during your early discussions with your oncologist, especially if you are of child-bearing age. A referral to a fertility specialist can provide more information and present you with options for what you can do. You may have the opportunity to preserve your eggs, or sperm, and consider alternate options for pregnancy in the future.

Intimacy

Cancer can, and often does, affect your life in ways you could never imagine. For the survivor trying to get his or her life on track, in all ways, you might find you need some time to slip back into normal patterns of behavior in your marriage, relationship, even dating . . . and by this, I do indeed mean you may have to make some post-cancer-treatment adjustments in your sex life.

As mentioned earlier, women undergoing a mastectomy or hysterectomy often experience body issues and psychological stress. A man undergoing a testicle removal can certainly feel some aftereffect that impinges on his feelings of masculinity. Fortunately, modern science can provide treatments and prosthetics to answer some of these concerns. What is harder to assuage is often a cancer patient's mental state. The idea of who we might have been before we had cancer and who we are now after our treatment, how we have changed in so many ways, can certainly leave one feeling less than confident. There is also the aftereffect, physical as well as mental, of exhaustion too many men and women feel after they have undergone months of worry and treatment over their cancer.

When you are sick, being intimate, even with the love of your life, can be the last thing on your mind.

Many cancer survivors report a loss of sexual interest, while just as many others see their desire increase now that they have survived something so horrific. Simply put, the question of intimacy comes to one and all on a case-by-case basis. If you are already part of a couple, it is sometimes easier to confront these changes, be they a muted libido or one supercharged, by discussing your feelings with your partner. Couples should know that plenty of counselors work in this area, and that often things can revert to what you were used to before cancer came calling. It is possible for both people to adjust well to what life has now presented them. As we know from even the most mundane concerns of our lives, our feelings are constantly morphing and changing. If we can just keep the communication open with our partner, we might find a new normal, even if it changes over time, very much to our liking.

The single person may have a more difficult time. Plenty of men and women are skittish indeed when experiencing their first intimate encounter post cancer treatment. If one sports some noticeable scar or dramatic change to their body, being seen naked by a new partner can be especially nerve-racking (although to be sure, if this is a new partner, they won't have any idea of what your body looked like before). If you feel a new relationship progressing to the point of it becoming sexual, communicating with your potential lover is essential. If your new partner does not know about your cancer by this point, the time to alert them is, quite frankly, now! If your fears are emotional and psychological more than physical, then yes, the discussion might be harder to have, but a revelation still needs to occur.

In almost every other aspect of our lives, worrying about something always presents the worst-case scenario we can think up. Usually, the reality we face is never as bad as the worst we can imagine. Secrets fester and grow, beyond natural proportions, the longer we keep them.

This certainly falls into the broad category of each person dealing with their personal life the best way they can. Be honest with your lover, be they your spouse of twenty years or someone you are getting to know better. All good sex comes from healthy communication; your intimate life after cancer should be no different.

Recurrence

But what happens to the survivor when cancer recurs? In some cases, having been through diagnosis and treatment already, a patient comes to their recurrence with more determination to get through the cancer treatment a second time; for many, it's the classic "devil you know" scenario. In other cases, people may have enjoyed years—even decades—cancer free, waiting for what they were convinced was the inevitable. Some are so completely surprised they have presented with cancer again that they simply give up all hope.

As Philip told us, he found two different mind-sets when it came to patients surviving longer with thankfully no signs of cancer recurrence: those who felt the longer they went cancer free the better their chances of staying cancer free, and those patients who, the longer they went, the more they felt the inevitable coming for them, as if cancer was waiting like a ticking bomb to present in them again the longer they went cancer free.

Unfortunately, recurrence does happen for some people, and I can't say with certainty what conclusion you will come to if your cancer does present again. But I can assure you, from my viewpoint, and as I said over and over, advances in science continue to make cancer treatment so much better, even if you were treated a mere few years ago. Do not give up hope. Do not simply surrender to that which you felt was inevitable. What you are either anticipating or might have some knowledge of, you will likely see is better now in some truly significant ways.

This is the good news.

The bad? Well, yes, there are some things about cancer treatment that don't change, and yes, you know the side effects are coming for you. But these can be battled as well by what we have learned in only a few short years, and your access to information now is such that you will be able to scour the web for people undergoing the exact treatment you are and reading how they are coming to survive it presently.

Good news again.

There are those cases where recurrence ends the life of the cancer patient. To this scenario I can only impart the advice I hope has been coming across loud and clear throughout all of this book . . . *live life to the fullest as much as you can every day you are alive*.

How Cultural Changes Have Shifted Views on Survivorship

As a scientist and as a cancer survivor, I wholeheartedly believe that the more information we have, the better. Also, the more information we have about surviving cancer, the more it leads to cultural changes. My own proactive measure to lessen my chances of acquiring breast cancer by insisting on surgery was met with resistance from my surgeon. As we learn more and more about long-term risks, preventive measures like the surgery I had, initially regarded as drastic or even unnecessary, will not be met with as much stigma and resistance.

Breast cancer, in general, is not stigmatized any longer. As our understanding of cancer grows, ignorance and misunderstanding retreat. Plenty of men present with breast cancer every year . . . and plenty survive it because the culture has changed in which, if a man feels a lump or pain in his chest, he won't so readily dismiss it as "a kind of cancer only women can get."

Through recent research and testing, the human papillomavirus (HPV to the layman) has been found and studied, and science has now developed a vaccine for it. While researchers initially discovered that this virus can cause cervical cancer in young women, we now also know that the virus is responsible for the development of other types of cancer, like head and neck cancer, which impact both women and men. HPV has been outed to such a degree that teenage girls and boys are both recommended to be vaccinated against it. While it's difficult to educate teenagers on the long-term implications, it is important for them to understand that without vaccination they could contract it themselves and possibly spread the virus to others in the future.

I feel that we are all a lot more comfortable speaking, thinking, and acting about cancer. This is as much from the research that has gone mainstream about the disease as it is from the fact that the more people who survive their cancer each day give us a living, breathing, active, and empowered population to learn from, live next to, love, and build our lives with.

One of the areas we might be lacking, though, where we have yet to catch up (although I know of people working in the field) is in the field of pediatric survivorship. Luckily, as with adults, many more kids are getting cancer free these days, and I know we will see a true cultural shift as we come to see more and more kids entering their teenage years and adulthood more cancer literate while being cancer free.

Survivorship for the Non-Patient

Grief, guilt, relief, depression, a call-to-action—I have no way of knowing how you are going to react as the caregiver surviving a loved one either dying from or being cured of cancer. I have seen a riot of emotions come down upon the survivor who is not the patient. I have seen families torn apart by cancer coming into their lives or rallying together. I have seen lovers grow strong as if going into battle to take down this disease that has come between them and a spouse as much as I have seen married couples simply give up, unable to face a loved one's decline. I have seen people work as hard as they can to make the final time as joyous as it can be, or completely collapse under the strain of impending death. Unfortunately, this all usually comes down to a know-it-when-I-get-there reality, something I wouldn't wish on anybody, of course. But if you have come to this book and this chapter specifically, I can assume some of these are your thoughts and concerns.

First and foremost, you must try and alleviate any guilt you are feeling. My dad and I could only do so much for my mom. As I told you, I did my best avoiding those deep talks about how long she had left, when I pretty much knew how long it would be; all the knowledge in the world does you little good when you are faced with a loved one who is suffering. I believe my mother and father made peace with my mother's cancer at the end, as much together as on their own. My dad grieved when she died. But my dad faced challenges after that, mostly getting used to a new normal in his everyday life.

My mother was the one who had paid the bills, so I had to get my dad up to speed on how to do that after my mother died. I was there about three times a week that first year, teaching him how to use the computer, going over paperwork with him, making sure he kept lawyer appointments and saw his financial planner. Luckily my dad has always been one of those guys who can cook for himself, do laundry, etc., so he didn't need help with these daily chores. But he did need to learn some tasks he simply had never done before. . . which he took to with aplomb.

I'm thrilled that my father feels as good as he does, mentally as well as physically. I have seen some long-married partners completely lose their way when a spouse dies, even dying soon after themselves.

Parents surviving their kids is a whole specific set of circumstances some people do not ever recover from. The people who meet LeAnn and are not aware of her background can be shocked to learn that such a get-up-and-go, with-it, fast-talking "sassy" lady has lived through such a tragedy in her life. She is one of the strong ones; she did manage to go on living. But I have seen plenty of parents who walk through the rest of their days like a zombie. I think we really should address the next subchapter with LeAnn specifically.

Parents Survivorship

Medulloblastoma is the most common brain tumor in children, meaning that there are about four to five hundred newly diagnosed cases each year in the United States, and it has a five-year survival rate of around 75% . . . although I do question those statistics. Although most of our 2008 was spent in and out of the hospital for my son's surgery/radiation/chemotherapy, and by that fall Cameron's treatment was complete. He was cancer free! He returned to school, our life returned to somewhat normal, and every three months we would return for scans. I became a determined mom to learn everything about cancer and his disease; surely if I was educated, I could make all the right decisions for his care for the rest of his life. This was survivorship 101 for us all, as far as I was concerned.

All was well until March 2010 when Cameron's two-year scan showed his cancer had returned to his spinal fluid. It was the classic out-of-body experience. Basically, I was going through my grief in survival mode. On the one hand I had been pleading with God to take my son, relieve him of his suffering, and when it finally happened I knew instantly he was in a better place. But at the same time, you suffer through terrible guilt; I was basically the worst mother in the world wishing that my son would die and being relieved suddenly that he was dead!

What I did was throw myself even deeper into patient advocacy and research. I was traveling to conferences, coming home, then going out again to speak at another meeting. My husband just didn't want to talk about Cameron's death; he kind of just hunkered down.

I generally have a very strong faith, but during that time I was pretty angry at God. Luckily, my faith was renewed after a time, and really it is only through the grace of God that our marriage survived. I know I could have become one of those parents who just give up, but I really believe I keep Cameron's beautiful spirit alive by doing what I do: fighting for patients' rights, participating in the conferences I do, helping people. He was the happiest, cutest kid, and I refuse to let cancer take any more of him from me, so I made a conscious decision to keep the conversation going about pediatric cancer care, to not carry a dark cloud over my head, to keep the fight going just like he would have wanted me to.

And that's how I survive.

⚜

It is certainly easier burying a parent than a child. When you see people with cancer passing in their eighties or nineties, their death is not as hard to take as someone cut down in the prime of their life by the disease.

Like Cameron. For many survivors who have attended a sick loved one, when that loved one dies, it becomes a matter of "what do I do now?" As I have mentioned, you can get consumed with attending to someone who is seriously ill. After that person dies, you can have a big space where you once had a clear-cut purpose. For other folks, and I had some of this with my father and his finances, simply doing things their partner used to do for them can offer strange everyday challenges.

Again, it's a matter of finding and adjusting to your new normal—this is a term Joyce uses as much as me. It really is the best way to describe your world before cancer came into it and your life after, no matter if you are patient or caregiver. I could lay out sentences of platitudes here, but I rather think rallying friends and family around you, as well as seeking professional help, will get you through those dark and debilitating feelings you might have surviving someone you love dying of cancer. In the resource section below, I list some places where to find this counseling.

Takeaways

- While the rate of cancer survivorship increases every day, this new paradigm of survivorship brings with it a whole host of concerns.
- Work with your doctor to create a survivorship plan, one that outlines what you've gone through and what lasting physical or mental symptoms you might have to manage.
- Those family members, friends, or caregivers who survive a cancer patient dying often need to adjust to a new normal as they continue without the patient.

RESOURCES:

ACS Cancer Survivors Network, https://csn.cancer.org/. As its name implies, this is an uplifting online depository of cancer survivors sharing their survival stories.

Bloch Cancer Foundation, http://blochcancer.org/, 1-800-433-0464, offers telephone matching to someone who is a survivor of your same type of cancer.

The Centers for Disease Control and Prevention, https://www.cdc.gov/cancer/survivorship/index.htm, presents this web portal specific to cancer survivorship.

ASCO Cancer.net, https://www.cancer.net/survivorship, provides doctor-approved information for cancer survivors.

The National Breast and Cervical Cancer Early Detection Program (NBCCEDP), https://www.cdc.gov/cancer/nbccedp/index.htm, is run by the Centers for Disease Control and Prevention (CDC) and is a source for low-income and uninsured women to find and facilitate breast and cervical cancer screenings.

The **National Coalition for Cancer Survivorship**, http://www.cancer-advocacy.org/, 1-877-622-7937 (toll free), again, offers a list of online publications on types of health insurance and coverage for those patients and caregivers who are attempting to surf the rough waters of finances in survivorship.

American Cancer Society's **Cancer Survivor's Network**, https://csn.cancer.org/. As you would expect, here is a far-reaching network of chat rooms and discussion boards, product reviews, and just about anything else survivors and their support group could need.

Conclusion

It's difficult to express how many people have come to me through the years with questions about their cancer. I wish I had all the answers to their questions and that the title of this book could be *Magic Bullet*, *Cure-All*, or *Panacea*.

It is not.

This book was always meant to be a practical primer for people who needed one. By sharing the knowledge and experience I have, I can hopefully alleviate someone else's suffering and maybe, in my own small way, add to the fight we are all undertaking to live with and eventually eradicate cancer. I hope that whatever brought you to these pages, you have a better understanding of the questions you need to ask and where to get your answers. But even beyond that, I hope that you know that you are not alone. And if my mom were still here today and asked me, "What about everyone who doesn't have someone like you? Who helps them when they have cancer?" I hope she would see this book as my answer.

I hope that you win your fight.

Detailed Resource Descriptions & Contact Information

Below are detailed descriptions of the sources I note from chapters two and onward, and some miscellaneous listings that don't appear in the book above. As you saw from the chapters, you might come to many of these sources for more than one concern.

Chapter 2: Building Your Healthcare Team

Certainly, one of the most reliable sources for cancer information is the American Cancer Society, https://www.cancer.org/, 1-800-ACS-2345 (toll free). You will find information at the ACS's website on types of cancer, diagnosis, treatment options, and so much more. Though I list this specific URL only once (but first!), you can assume that no matter your concern, in almost all of the categories below, the AMS can either directly help you or be able to refer you to a source that can. You will see where I list other specific pages from them later.

Healthgrades' **National Health Index**, https://www.healthgrades.com/. Twenty-five U.S. cities exist in their network for connecting patients, healthcare providers, and hospitals.

U Compare Healthcare, http://www.ucomparehealthcare.com/, provides net-based tools for anyone looking to compare the various healthcare services available.

The **National Center for Biotechnology Information** (NBI), https://www.ncbi.nlm.nih.gov/, is a sprawling government website full of information on all aspects of human health. Tending toward hard scientific research, the web pages are not always so easy to get through, but there is invaluable information here on almost every aspect of what to be looking for in your healthcare.

American Society of Clinical Oncology's Cancer.Net, http://www.cancer. net, provides doctor-approved information for cancer patients, and offers suggestions on how to navigate your cancer diagnosis and care.

Chapter 3: What Type of Cancer Do I Have?

The **American Cancer Society**, https://www.cancer.org/, 1-800-ACS-2345 (toll free).

The **National Breast and Cervical Cancer Early Detection Program (NBCCEDP)**, https://www.cdc.gov/cancer/nbccedp/index.htm, helps low-income and uninsured women to find and facilitate breast and cervical cancer screenings.

The **National Cancer Institute** (NHI), https://www.cancer.gov/, proclaims it is "the nation's leader in cancer research." It provides a deep well of information.

Cancer Treatment Centers of America (CTCA), https://www.cancercenter. com/, 855-412-1358, has constantly updated blog posts, research on treatment and cancer types, and so many other concerns for patients and caregiver. Treatment, insurance, options for metastatic brain tumors, and much more information is available at this site.

The **Leukemia and Lymphoma Society**, www.lls.org, 1-800-955-4572.

For patients with leukemia, lymphoma, or myeloma, the LLS offers assistance on services and treatments, transportation to treatment centers, and financial assistance for insurance co-payments. They have chapters in fifty states.

The **Cancer Support Community**, https://www.cancersupportcommunity.org/, 888-793-9355, (toll free). Like the AMS, the CSC offers a multi–web page resource for the many questions you might have about cancer and where to find support.

The **National Cancer Institutes' Seer Training Modules**, https://training.seer.cancer.gov, are an invaluable resource of web pages about all aspects of cancer.

The **National Comprehensive Cancer Network**, https://www.nccn.org/, is another invaluable resource for fighting cancer.

American Society of Clinical Oncology's Cancer.Net, http://www.cancer.net, provides doctor-approved information for cancer patients, and offers suggestions on how to navigate your cancer diagnosis and care.

Counseling & Emotional Support

The **CancerCare Organization**, https://www.cancercare.org/, 1-800-813-HOPE, offers face-to-face, online, and telephone counseling for a multitude of concerns. They provide counseling, support groups, education, and even financial assistance.

The **American Psychosocial Oncology Society**, https://apos-society.org/, 1-866-276-7443, offers telephone referrals for counseling. Begun in 1986 to connect people working in the psychological, behavioral, and social concerns of cancer, as of the beginning of the century the APOS has bolstered their network to now include professionals in all the disciplines of psychosocial oncology. Counselors to clergy to all level of people working in the psychological and social sciences can be found here.

Cancer Information and Counseling Line, http://amc.org.s104393. gridserver.com/programs.html, 1-800-525-3777 (an affiliate of AMC Cancer Research Center). Another deep resource you will see me listing often here offers telephone counseling to cancer patients and their families.

Chapter 4: Treatment

The **National Cancer Institute**'s specific page on cancer treatment, https:// www.cancer.gov/about-cancer/treatment, 1-800-4-cancer. Here the NIH lays out information of cancer types and their specific treatments, lists of side effects, and an A–Z rundown of cancer drugs. CAMS are even explained here.

American Cancer Society's specific page on cancer treatment, https:// www.cancer.org/treatment/treatments-and-side-effects/treatment-types. html, 800-227-2345. Every bit as extensive as the NIH's page.

Natural Medicines Comprehensive Database, www.naturalmedicines-database.com, provides the largest number of evidence-based reviews. Authors are primarily doctors of pharmacy. Includes scientific names, uses, safety, effectiveness, mechanism of action, adverse reactions, interactions, and dosage.

Complementary and Alternative Medicines (CAMS)

American Cancer Society's specific page on alternate treatments, https:// www.cancer.org/treatment/treatments-and-side-effects/complementary-and-alternative-medicine.html.

National Center for Complementary and Alternative Medicine, www. nccam.nih.gov. This is the U.S. government's lead agency for scientific research on CAM. The NCCAM's mission is to define, through rigorous scientific investigation, the usefulness and safety of CAM interventions and their roles in improving health and healthcare. Includes review of scientific evidence for usefulness, toxicities, and precautions.

Cam-Cancer, http://www.cam-cancer.org/, is an "open-access, nonprofit web resource" for health professionals looking to gaining further information and assist in treatment options via CAM care.

Chapter 5: So You Want to Participate in a Clinical Trial

ACS's **Clinical Trial Matching Service**, https://www.cancer.org/treatment/ treatments-and-side-effects/clinical-trials/clinical-trials-matching-service-find-trial.html, 800-303-5691, offers a free, confidential program to help patients, their families, and healthcare workers find cancer clinical trials most appropriate for a patient's medical and personal situation.

The **National Cancer Institute**'s page on clinical trials, https://www.cancer. gov/about-cancer/treatment/clinical-trials/patient-safety/childrens-assent. A vast resource of every facet of clinical trials. Here the NCI also provides a section on the specific of pediatric clinical trials.

The **Food and Drug Administration**'s site for informed consent for clinical trials: https://www.fda.gov/ForPatients/ClinicalTrials/InformedConsent/ default.htm.

The **U. S. National Library of Medicine** site, http://www.ClinicalTrials. gov, is both privately and publicly funded. This database lists the multiple clinical trials patients can participate it, broken down by types of cancer being tested and other specific criteria.

Chapter 6: The Business of Your Health—Health Insurance, Legal

Patient Advocate Foundation (PAF), www.patientadvocate.org, 800-532-5274. In addition to the work they do with advocacy, they also offer a Co-Pay Relief Program, which provides financial assistance to patients.

This is the **National Coalition for Cancer Survivorship** URL and toll-free phone number, http://www.canceradvocacy.org/, 1-877-622-7937. The NCCS offers a list of online publications that explore the many types of health insurance and health coverage.

The Employee Benefits Security Administration at the U.S. Department of Labor, https://www.dol.gov/agencies/ebsa, can help you explore your employer's health plan particulars as well as answer any other questions concerning the law and your employee rights.

The Hill-Burton Program, available in all states except IN, NE, NV, RI, UT, or WY, offers reduced-cost healthcare services to patients who prove eligible. They can be reached by calling 1-800-638-0742.

The **National Breast and Cervical Cancer Early Detection Program** (NBCCEDP) runs such a program in conjunction with the Centers for Disease Control and Prevention (CDC), offers low-income, the uninsured, and many other women the opportunity for breast and cervical cancer screening. Find them here: https://www.cdc.gov/cancer/nbccedp/index.htm.

The **Cancer Legal Resource Center Cancer Legal Resource Center Hotline** (at 866-THE-CLRC) matches cancer patients and survivors to volunteer attorneys. The CLRC can also provide information and resources on cancer-related legal issues and general legal advice.

As mentioned previously, the **Leukemia and Lymphoma Society** is not only one of the best resources for patients with leukemia, lymphoma, or myeloma, it also offers assistance for services, treatments, transportation, and financial assistance for the insured's co-pays.

The **FMLA** can be reached here: (866) 487-9243 or (887) 889-5827 and at www.dol.gov/esa/whd/fmla.

Find out all you need to know about **HIPAA** (and plenty of other healthcare related laws) here: https://www.hhs.gov/hipaa/for-individuals/guidance-materials-for-consumers/index.html.

The Partnership for Prescription Assistance (PPA), 888-477-2669, www.pparx.org, offers nearly five hundred programs for low-cost and free prescription drugs for millions of Americans, with two hundred offered by biopharmaceutical companies.

The Social Security Administration website, for any and all concerns about employment, can be found here: https://www.ssa.gov/disability/.

The Employee Benefits Security Administration at the U.S. Department of Labor, again to answer questions of employment and worker's rights, can be found here: https://www.dol.gov/agencies/ebsa.

Chapter 7: So, You Are the Caregiver

The American Cancer Society's **Caregivers and Family** website, https://www.cancer.org/treatment/caregivers.html, 800-277-2345, is a full resource for what caregivers can come to expect. As with most ACS pages, there really isn't any stone left unturned here in information and resources for the people who come to care for the cancer patient.

The Caregiver Action Network, https://www.cancersupportcommunity.org/caregivers, is a web portal cancer support community for caregivers. Practical advice here is offered for a patient's cancer protocols and exactly what a caregiver should be concerning themselves with, as well as how to address these issues.

The **Cancer Net**, https://www.cancer.net/coping-with-cancer/caring-loved-one, is a web portal specifically designed for caregivers. Here visitors will get doctor-approved advice from the American Society of Clinical Oncology.

Share the Caregiving Inc., https://sharethecare.org/, is a not-for-profit program developed from the National Center for Civic Innovation, and based on the STC guidebook. Published in 1995, here caregivers can find information and suggestions on maintaining their efforts, even over a long period.

Caring Bridge Network, https://www.caringbridge.org, is a massive social network designed for cancer patients and their caregivers, friends, and family to communicate via modern technology and the vast resources of social media.

Advocacy

Patient Advocate Foundation (PAF), www.patientadvocate.org, 800-532-5274, offers assistance to both insured and uninsured patients, helping in coordinating benefits managing of cases. Here one can find help in arbitration, mediation, and any other aspect of settling issues related to the legal aspects of a patient's cancer care.

The AdvoConnection Directory, https://advoconnection.com/. Patients and private advocates connect here to navigate both the U.S. and Canada's oftentimes complicated healthcare system.

Values Based Patient Advocates, https://valuesbasedpa.com/, (703) 222-1300. The massive listing here are of advocates who are 100% unbiased.

Full information is provided through contacts for whatever disease a patient has and the treatments they might come to face.

Chapter 8: End of Life Decisions

National Hospice and Palliative Care Organization Caring Connections, 800-658-8898, http://www.caringinfo.org/i4a/pages/index.cfm?pageid=1, offers all levels of advice and free resources for people coming to end-of-life decisions. Supported by all kinds of funding to the NHF.

The **American Hospice Foundation (AHF)**, https://americanhospice.org/, closed in June 2014, but you can still find here a wealth of information about hospice. A legacy library left for furthering hospice care through public education, professional training, and consumer advocacy.

The **National Cancer Institute**, https://www.cancer.gov/about-cancer/advanced-cancer/care-choices/care-fact-sheet, a webpage for end-of-life care run by the National Cancer Institute.

The **American Cancer Society**, https://www.cancer.org/treatment/end-of-life-care/nearing-the-end-of-life.html. The massive portal for end-of-life-care from the equally massive ACS.

The **National Association for Home Care & Hospice (NAHC)**, https://www.nahc.org/, web page for the trade association of resources, education, and advocacy for hospice and the people who need it. The NAHC is nonprofit, representing the U.S.'s 33,000 home care and hospice organizations. It also advocates for over two million nurses, therapists, and aides.

Caring Connections of the National Hospice and Palliative Care Organization, http://www.caringinfo.org/i4a/pages/index.cfm?pageid=3289, 800-658-8898. Here patients and caregivers can find a downloadable PDF applicable for each U.S. state cancer care and hospice. Although the materials are copyrighted, permission is granted to download a single copy of any portion of the text.

Chapter 9: How to Survive Surviving Cancer

ACS's **Cancer Survivors Network,** https://csn.cancer.org/, As its name implies, this is an uplifting online depository of cancer survivors sharing their survival stories. Discussion boards, a chat room, resource library, and updated announcements are just some of what is offered here.

Bloch Cancer Foundation, http://blochcancer.org/, 1-800-433-0464, offers telephone matching to someone who is a survivor of your same type of cancer.

The Centers for Disease Control and Prevention, https://www.cdc. gov/cancer/survivorship/index.htm, presents this web portal specific to cancer survivorship. Here you will find cancer survivor stories, resources, and basic information for cancer survivors, their families, and healthcare professionals.

ASCO Cancer.net, https://www.cancer.net/survivorship, provides doctor-approved information for cancer survivors. Here you can find survivorship resources, facts on the long-term side effects of cancer treatment, learn about pregnancy post cancer, and even find artwork by survivors.

The **National Breast and Cervical Cancer Early Detection Program (NBCCEDP),** https://www.cdc.gov/cancer/nbccedp/index.htm, run by the Centers for Disease Control and Prevention (CDC), and source for low-income and uninsured women to find and facilitate breast and cervical cancer screenings. As I have mentioned, the ways in which we can facilitate early detection presently saves lives!

The **National Coalition for Cancer Survivorship**, http://www.cancer-advocacy.org/, 1-877-622-7937 (toll free), again, offers a list of online publications on types of health insurance and coverage for those patients and caregivers who are attempting to surf the rough waters of finances in survivorship.

American Cancer Society's **Cancer Survivor's Network**, https://csn.cancer.org/. As you would expect, here is a far-reaching network of chat rooms and discussion boards, product reviews, and nearly anything else survivors and their support group could need.

www.ingramcontent.com/pod-product-compliance
Lightning Source LLC
Chambersburg PA
CBHW072139270326
41931CB00010B/1806